Save Your Aching Back and Neck
A Patient's Guide

Second Edition

Authors
Stewart G. Eidelson, M.D.
Richard G. Fessler, M.D., Ph.D.
Steven R. Garfin, M.D.
Steven H. Richeimer, M.D.
Gerald E. Rodts, Jr., M.D.
Susan A. Spinasanta

Contributors
Christopher M. Bono, M.D.
Dana L. Davis, M.P.T., M.T.T.
Gregory Gilreath, P.A.-C.
Robert E. Isaacs, M.D.
Laurie Morse, L.Ac., Q.M.E.
Laurie Rice-Wyllie, R.N., M.S., A.N.P.C.
Gerardo Zloczover, M.D.

Editor
Stewart G. Eidelson, M.D.

Publisher
SYA Press and Research, Inc.

Save Your Aching Back and Neck
A Patient's Guide - Second Edition

Disclaimer:

Published by:
SYA Press and Research, Inc.
5694 Mission Center Road #294
San Diego, CA 92108-4380
(561) 995-1437
books@spineuniverse.com

Copyright © 2002 SYA Press and Research, Inc.
Printed in the United States of America
ISBN   09669252-1-1
First printing: April 1999
Second printing: May 2002, completely revised

Library of Congress Cataloging-in-Publication Data

Eidelson, M.D., Stewart G.
Fessler, M.D., Ph.D., Richard G.
Garfin, M.D., Steven R.
Richeimer, M.D., Steven H.
Rodts, Jr., M.D., Gerald E.
Spinasanta, Susan A.

Includes biographical references, illustrations, and index.

Dedications

To My Mother, Diana Burger

A loving mother and friend whose energy and unyielding support has been a guiding light for my personal success.

To Ed Traurig

A rare "genius" for recognizing and supporting endeavers driven by individual passion. The publication of *Save Your Aching Back...A Patient's Guide* and the development of *spineuniverse.com* is a direct result of Ed's personal commitment and encouragement to a friend.

Acknowledgements

If you have ever set out to write a book, you know it is a difficult proposition. It is only with a great deal of help from others that a book becomes published and successful. *Save Your Aching Back and Neck, A Patient's Guide* is no exception.

Some of the finest medical specialists have taken from their valuable time to contribute chapters to this book. Our gratitude for their fine work cannot be put into words worthy of our appreciation.

Richard G. Fessler, M.D., Ph.D. with assistance from his Spine Fellow, Robert E. Isaacs, M.D., and Laurie Rice-Wyllie, R.N., M.S., A.N.P.C. provides a patient's perspective of minimally invasive spine surgery for treatment of a lumbar herniated disc.

Steven R. Garfin, M.D. and his Spine Fellow Christopher M. Bono, M.D. present a chapter about degenerative changes affecting the cervical spine and options for treatment.

Steven H. Richeimer, M.D. provides an entire chapter about pain and how it can be managed.

Gerald E. Rodts, Jr., M.D. gives us insight into the future of spine surgery, trends, and the Internet.

Susan A. Spinasanta was instrumental in organizing and overseeing the work to produce this book. Not only did she rewrite and update most chapters from the previous edition, *Save Your Aching Back, A Patient's Guide*, but also worked with each contributing author through the submission and editorial processes.

Dana L. Davis, M.P.T., M.T.T. outlines the positive aspects of physical therapy and the benefits.

Gregory Gilreath, P.A.-C., who treats patients with spine disorders every day, summarizes what patients need to know before spine surgery.

Laurie Morse, L.Ac., Q.M.E. presents valuable information about acupuncture and other types of Traditional Chinese Medicine from which so many patients have benefitted.

Gerardo Zloczover, M.D. presents excellent information about the integrated approach to back and neck pain.

We would also like to thank *spineuniverse.com* for permission to use their excellent anatomical illustrations. It is hoped that these illustrations will serve our readers well.

Biographies

Stewart G. Eidelson, M.D. is an Orthopaedic Spine Surgeon with offices in Boca Raton and Boynton Beach, FL. He is the Founder of *spineuniverse.com*, the most comprehensive website dedicated to the spine.

After graduation from Drew University in Madison, NJ, he attended Thomas Jefferson Medical College in Philadelphia, PA. Following graduation in 1976, he completed his internship at Metropolitan Hospital in New York.

Dr. Eidelson completed his orthopaedic residences at the Geisinger Medical Center in Danville, PA and the Alfred I. duPont Institute in Wilmington, DE. Later, he trained under the direction of Dr. Arthur Steffee in spine surgery at the Cleveland Spine Center.

Dr. Eidelson is a member of the North American Spine Society, the Palm Beach County Medical Society, the Florida Orthopaedic Society, and the Palm Beach County Orthopaedic Society. He is Board Certified by the American Board of Orthopaedic Surgery and is a Fellow of the American Academy of Orthopaedic Surgeons.

Further, Dr. Eidelson has a keen interest in outcome studies relating to spinal surgical procedures performed on elderly patients. In conjunction with this important research, many of his papers have been accepted and presented worldwide.

At the community level, in addition to a large spine care nonsurgical and surgical practice, Dr. Eidelson presents seminars to educate the public about spinal anatomy, disorders, and treatment options.

Stewart G. Eidelson, M.D.

Richard G. Fessler, M.D., Ph.D. is a Neurosurgeon. He is the Founder and Director of the Institute for Spine Care at the Chicago Institute of Neurosurgery and Neuroresearch (CINN) and is a Professor of Neurological Surgery at Rush Medical School in Chicago, IL.

At the University of Chicago, Dr. Fessler completed with honors a Medical Doctorate, and Surgical and Neurosurgical residences. In addition to surgical training, he completed a Doctorate of Philosophy in Pharmacology and Physiology. Dr. Fessler held research Fellowships at the University of Chicago Medical Center in Neurological Surgery and Psychiatry. The Chicago Surgical Society honored Dr. Fessler with the Excellence in Surgical Research award.

Dr. Fessler has made significant contributions to the development of minimally invasive spine surgery. The Kambin Foundation awarded Dr. Fessler the annual research award for his work in this field.

He is a member of the American Medical Association, Congress of Neurological Surgeons, American Association of Neurological Surgeons, Neurological Society of America, Joint Section on Disorders of the Spine and Peripheral Nerves, North American Skull Base Society, Joint Section on Pain, Joint Section on Trauma and Critical Care, American College of Surgeons, Society of Neurological Surgeons, Southern Neurosurgical Society, and the North American Spine Society. In several of these professional organizations Dr. Fessler has held leadership positions.

In addition, Dr. Fessler is currently on Advisory Committees for the Food and Drug Administration and has served on government committees of the Department of Health and Human Services and the National Head Injury Foundation. (Continued)

Richard G. Fessler, M.D., Ph.D.

He is a prolific author and lends his expertise to the Editorial Boards of *Neurosurgery* and *Neuro-Orthopaedics*. Three times he has been listed among the *Best Doctors in America* and is a Medical Specialist and Flight Surgeon for NASA/Space Shuttle.

Steven R. Garfin, M.D. is an Orthopaedic Surgeon, and Professor and Chairman of the Department of Orthopaedics at the University of California.

Dr. Garfin earned a Medical Degree at the University of Minnesota and was honored with the Alpha Omega Alpha Society award. He completed his internship in Surgery and residency in Orthopaedic Surgery at the University of California, San Diego. As an orthopaedic resident, Dr. Garfin received the Zimmer-McCoy Residency Award and the Alfred V. Bateman Resident Anatomy Award. Under direction of Doctors R. H. Rothman and F. A. Simeone, Dr. Garfin received Fellowship training in Disorders of the Spine at Pennsylvania Hospital.

Since his Fellowship, Dr. Garfin has received numerous awards such as the Volvo Award for Research (twice), AcroMed Research Award of the North American Spine Society (three times), the Cervical Spine Research Society Research Award (twice), and the Orthopaedic Research Society New Investigator Recognition Award. More recently, the North American Spine Society awarded Dr. Garfin the Wiltse Award for Leadership in the Field of Spine.

Dr. Garfin is a member of the Academic Orthopaedic Society, American Academy of Orthopaedic Surgeons, American Orthopaedic Association, Cervical Spine Research Society, International Society for the Study of the Lumbar Spine, North American Spine Society, and the Orthopaedic Research Society. For several of

Steven R. Garfin, M.D.

these societies Dr. Garfin has held leadership positions including President, Board Member, and Program Chairman.

In addition, Dr. Garfin's impressive published research and writing include many books, book chapters, peer-reviewed journal articles and abstracts. Currently Dr. Garfin is a Deputy Editor of *Spine* and Reviewer for the *Journal of Orthopaedic Research, Journal of American Medical Association, Clinical Orthopaedics and Related Research*, and *Journal of Bone and Joint Surgery*.

Steven H. Richeimer, M.D. is Associate Professor of Anesthesiology and Psychiatry at the University of Southern California at Davis. He is also the Director of USC Pain Management and Director, Norris Cancer Hospital Pain Management. Dr. Richeimer is Board Certified in the fields of Anesthesiology and Psychiatry, and in the sub-specialty of Pain Management.

Dr. Richeimer earned a Medical Degree from the University of California San Francisco School of Medicine. He completed residencies at the University of California Los Angeles in anesthesiology and psychiatry. Dr. Richeimer completed pain management training at Harvard's Beth Israel Hospital in Boston, MA.

At the University of California Davis Medical Center he established a national reputation for his comprehensive and multidisciplinary approach to pain management.

Dr. Richeimer is a member of the American Pain Society, American Society of Regional Anesthesia, American Society of Anesthesiologists, International Association for the Study of Pain, and the American Medical Association.

Steven H. Richeimer, M.D.

Gerald E. Rodts, Jr., M.D. is a Neurosurgeon. He is an Associate Professor of Neurosurgery and Co-Director of the Spine Fellowship for the Department of Neurosurgery at Emory University School of Medicine. He is Director of the Emory NeuroSpine Institute in Atlanta, GA.

Dr. Rodts completed his Medical Degree at Columbia University. At the University of California Los Angeles School of Medicine he trained as an intern in General Surgery and a resident in Neurological Surgery. At Emory University he was a Fellow in Spinal Neurosurgery.

Currently, Dr. Rodts is Secretary for the Congress of Neurological Surgeons (CNS) and Treasurer for the American Association of Neurological Surgeons (AANS) and the Congress of Neurological Surgeons' Joint Section on Disorders of the Spine and Peripheral Nerves. Dr. Rodts is a member of the Congress of Neurological Surgeons, American Association of Neurological Surgeons, AANS-CNS Joint Section on Disorders of the Spine and Peripheral Nerves, and the Southern Neurological Society.

Dr. Rodts has published many articles in peer-reviewed journals, contributed chapters to medical textbooks, and presented numerous papers and posters at worldwide professional meetings highlighting his research in minimally invasive spine surgery and computer-assisted image-guided spine surgery.

Gerald E. Rodts, Jr., M.D.

Susan A. Spinasanta is the Manager, Content Development for *spineuniverse.com*. She is a writer and editor with expertise in spinal orthopaedics, spine surgery, neurology, neurosurgery, and general medicine. She has written and edited books and journal articles for publication. Ms. Spinasanta's experience includes clinical trials, scientific papers (petrochemical), process control, and technical manuals for computerized manufacturing systems.

Christopher M. Bono, M.D. is an Orthopaedic Surgeon. He is Fellowship trained in Spine Surgery under Steven R. Garfin, M.D. at the University of California at San Diego. Dr. Bono earned a Medical Degree at SUNY Health Science Center at Brooklyn, NY. He completed his Orthopaedic Residency at NJ Medical School, Department of Orthopaedics, University of Medicine and Dentistry of New Jersey in Newark, NJ.

In addition, Dr. Bono received the following honors: 2000 Resident Research and 2000 Resident Teaching Awards, 1999 Excellence Award, and 1998 Resident Research Award from the New Jersey Medical School, Department of Orthopaedics. Dr. Bono's published research includes many peer-reviewed articles, book chapters, and presentations.

Dana L. Davis, M.P.T., M.T.T received a Master's of Physical Therapy from the Institute of Physical Therapy at St. Augustine, FL. Her professional strengths include manual therapy, wound care, sports orthopaedics, back and neck dysfunction, and management. In addition, Ms. Davis' professional experience includes patient treatment in different settings; rehabilitation facilities, hospital, outpatient, and nursing.

Gregory Gilreath, P.A.-C. is Physician's Assistant to Stewart G. Eidelson, M.D. He has more than 40 years of medical experience, 30 years of which has been dedicated to orthopaedic spine surgery. A former native of Cincinnati, OH and graduate of the University of Cincinnati, Mr. Gilreath received degrees in zoology, psychology, and surgical assisting technology. At the Mayfield Neurological Institute in Cincinnati, he was trained in neurological procedures. Mr. Gilreath also trained and functioned with the U.S. Army Medical Corps.

Further, Mr. Gilreath trained under several noteworthy spine specialists such as Arthur Steffee, M.D., John Collis, M.D., Charles Edwards, M.D., Gabriel Ma, M.D., and Ralph Cloward, M.D. (one of the founding "Fathers" of spinal surgery).

Robert E. Isaacs, M.D. received his medical degree from Baylor College of Medicine in Houston, TX. At Baylor he received several awards including Doctor of Medicine with Honors, Presidential Scholar, Honors in the Basic Sciences, and Outstanding Performance in Clinical Neurology. Dr. Isaacs completed his surgical internship and neurosurgical residency at Vanderbilt University in Nashville, TN. He received neurological training at Barrow Neurological Institute in Phoenix, AZ.

Dr. Isaacs is currently completing a clinical spine Fellowship under Richard G. Fessler, M.D., Ph.D. at the Chicago Institute of Neurosurgery and Neuroresearch (CINN) through Rush University in Chicago, IL.

Laurie Morse, L.Ac., Q.M.E. is an Acupuncturist. Ms. Morse received a Master's Degree in Traditional Oriental Medicine from the Pacific College of Oriental Medicine in San Diego, CA. She is a Licensed and Board Certified Acupuncturist.

Ms. Morse is a native of Southern California and began studying holistic medicine more than 15 years ago. She has a rich knowledge of Chinese Medicine including Chinese Herbs, nutrition, massage, aromatherapy, meditation, and guided imagery. Her areas of interest using Traditional Chinese Medicine include pain management, stress management, women's health, digestive disorders, and preventive health maintenance.

Laurie Rice-Wyllie, R.N., M.S., A.N.P.C. is a microsurgical nurse practitioner with over ten years of neurosurgery experience. She currently works with Richard Fessler, M.D., Ph.D., a neurosurgeon with the Chicago Institute of Neurosurgery and Neuroresearch (CINN).

Ms. Rice-Wyllie began her nursing education at Indiana University and completed her Master and Nurse Practitioner degrees at Loyola University at Chicago, IL. She is an author, lecturer, and researcher.

Gerardo Zloczover, M.D. specializes in anesthesiology. He graduated from Universidad Peruana Cayetano Heredia, Lima, Peru. His internship was performed at Baltimore City Hospital and he completed his residency at the University of Miami. He is a Diplomate of the American Board of Anesthesiology and has been in private practice since 1982.

Table of Contents

Introduction

Chapters

Table of Contents

Introduction

Stewart G. Eidelson, M.D.

During my 18 years as a practicing surgeon treating thousands of patients, I have learned that the average person doesn't know where to start to find out about their condition and available treatment options. In addition to obtaining trustworthy information, I have found that each patient needs to analyze and evaluate his or her options.

Many daily decisions are easy, comfortable, and may be based on what has been learned or what may feel instinctively correct. However, most people, whether they are the patient or the caregiver, may find making healthcare decisions an uneasy and difficult experience.

There are many components to making a healthcare decision. Some things to consider include the diagnosis, necessity of a second opinion, nonsurgical and surgical treatment options, long and short term effects of treatment, patient preferences, and of course, the risks. To these components add medical jargon and it is easy to see why making these types of decisions can be frustrating and even disappointing.

To help people understand the spine, aging, and degenerative conditions, diseases, diagnostic tests, nonsurgical treatment and surgical procedures, as well as new technological advances, I started to present public forums many years ago. At each forum a different topic about the spine is presented. In addition, the audience is encouraged to participate during a lengthy question and answer session. The forums have proven to be enlightening not only to the attendees but also myself.

Introduction

I recognized the need for a practical and easy to read book for patients about the spine. This led to writing *Save Your Aching Back, A Patient's Guide* published in 1999. The book proved to be a hit with patients and others interested in spinal disorders, surgery, and other related topics.

The positive feedback from readers began to pour in and it wasn't long until I realized a second edition was needed. It was at this time that I founded *spineuniverse.com*, an extensive website dedicated to bringing the best minds and technology together on the subject of back and neck pain. At *spineuniverse.com* people can post their questions about the spine that are answered on line by a spine expert. This proved to be another valuable resource to determine what patients want to know.

So that leads us to the book you have in your hand – *Save Your Aching Back and Neck, A Patient's Guide*. This edition is a compendium written by some of the leaders in the spine field and addresses not only the back, but also the neck. Yet this comprehensive book is still small enough to be carried in a pocket or purse.

You will find the revised anatomy chapter is filled with new illustrations to help you understand the elements of the spine. In addition, there are many new chapters that include minimally invasive low back surgery, neck disorders and treatment, pain management, the future of spine surgery, the Internet, physical therapy, and even Traditional Chinese Medicine.

• Richard G. Fessler, M.D., Ph.D., a distinguished neurosurgeon, and Founder and Director of the Institute for Spine Care at the Chicago Institute of Neurosurgery and Neuroresearch (CINN) discusses the lumbar spine and minimally invasive spine surgery.

• A new chapter about common cervical disorders and treatment has been written by Steven R. Garfin, M.D., Professor and Chairman of the Department of Orthopaedics, Spine Surgery, at UCSD School of Medicine.

• Doctor Steven H. Richeimer, is Director of USC at Davis Pain Management, and Associate Professor of Anesthesiology and Psychiatry. He provides an excellent chapter about pain management and strategies used to control pain.

• New advancements in spine surgery and its future, as well as the advantages the Internet offers patients today is provided by Gerald E. Rodts, Jr., M.D., Associate Professor and Co-Director of the Spine Fellowship for the Department of Neurosurgery at Emory University School of Medicine.

• Dana L. Davis, M.P.T., M.T.T. answers common questions patients ask about physical therapy.

• Laurie Morse, L.Ac., QME discusses acupuncture and Traditional Chinese Medicine in relationship to back pain.

• Gerardo Zloczover, M.D. discusses the integrated treatment approach to spine pain.

• Plus – the glossary has been expanded!

I hope you will find *Save Your Aching Back and Neck, A Patient's Guide* practical and easy to use. Your comments are always welcome.

Speaking for all the authors, we hope you find this book as helpful as the authors found it enjoyable to assemble for your benefit.

Introduction

Chapter 1

Seniors — You Are Not Alone!

Like many people their age, Joe and Lillian vacation in Florida during the cold winter months. During their drive south Joe daydreams about golf and improving his handicap. As soon as they arrive at their destination Joe quickly unloads the car and soon finds himself on the golf course with friends. Later that evening Joe's lower back begins to ache and feel stiff. He brushes the pain off as simply the price paid for a near perfect game of golf. Several days pass and Joe is beginning to wonder why his back *still* aches.

Does Joe's problem sound familiar? Fortunately, Joe's problem was not serious. What happened to him commonly affects millions of people each year. He had not been golfing for a couple of months. His back muscles were not conditioned to repeatedly swing a golf club. Joe's case is an example why back pain is so prevalent in America. At any given time 80% of the adult population in the United States may be affected by a back or neck disorder.

Human beings have many things in common that play important roles in the health of the spine. Heredity is an example. Scoliosis (sko-lee-oh-sis) is a spinal disorder that may run in families. This disease causes the spine to curve abnormally to one side ("S" or "C" shaped curve). When diagnosed early, steps can be taken to help control scoliosis. Individual family trees may reveal clues to future health. This is why the physician asks about family history.

The process of normal aging affects the spine and may lead to degenerative disorders. Unfortunately there is no magic pill or treatment to stop this natural process although heredity may lend a clue to longevity. If your parents and grandparents lived long lives and you inherited those good genes you may live longer too. However living longer does not guarantee quality of life because the affects from fighting gravity may be more pronounced in some people.

The number of older Americans is growing. People of all ages are looking for ways to prolong life, stay healthy and remain active. Today attitudes about aging and activity are changing. It is not unusual to read about older people participating in the Olympics, triathlons, tennis, and other competitive sports.

Improved public health has helped to increase longevity. For example, the toxicity (poison) caused by smoking and tobacco products is well-known. Smokers are less healthy than non-smokers and are at a greater risk for spine problems (i.e. osteoporosis). Today scientists know that certain chemical toxins can alter the genetic code that could affect future generations.

Medicines have been developed to help control diseases that at one time may have meant certain death. The quality of life for people afflicted with a spinal disorder continues to improve. New technology and other advancements have made it possible to perform complex spinal surgery on children, adults and seniors.

The importance of maintaining a healthy weight and regular exercise is proven. Obesity causes unnecessary stress to the spine and cardiovascular system.

The spine was designed for activity. The muscles in the spine need to be conditioned and strong to help support the vertebral (ver-tee-brawl) column. This is one reason why physical therapy may be incorporated into a patient's treatment plan.

The goal of physical therapy is to restore the patient's functional ability so they can return to golf, swimming, walking, and other activities. Muscle conditioning and exercise help muscles to be strong enough to meet the physical challenges of everyday life.

There is not a fountain of youth or a magic pill to keep our bodies free from the effects of aging. However, we can regularly exercise and eat well each day as a part of a healthier lifestyle.

The following chapter is about the anatomy of the spine. Learn about the bones, discs, ligaments, muscles, and nerves in the spine and how they function. This information may help you to understand spinal disorders, treatments, and how lifestyle choices may help you to prevent spine problems.

Chapter 2

The Spine:
An Integral Part of the Human Body

The purpose of this chapter is to introduce you to the human spine. As part of the body, the spine is a unique and complex structure. The spine is composed of living bone, cartilaginous elements (car-t-lay-gin-us), joints, a spinal cord, nerve roots, ligaments, tendons, muscles, and a vascular system. The whole body, as well as the spine, is dependent on the function of each element. Knowledge about these spinal elements may help you to better understand how lifestyle, aging, injury, and disease may adversely affect the spine.

The **Human Skeleton** is the body's framework or scaffolding system. Skeletal bones are classified as long, short, flat, or irregular and vary in length, width, and depth. The bones in the spine are irregular in shape and provide places to connect to other bones. The function of the skeletal system is to support the body against the force of gravity, protect soft body parts, produce red blood cells, store inorganic calcium, and phosphorus salts, and to provide sites for muscle attachment to enable body movement.

Bone is a living tissue. During prenatal development bones are cartilaginous. A newborn's body may contain more than 300 cartilaginous bones that gradually fuse to form approximately 206 permanent bones by adulthood. Osteoblasts (os-t-o-blasts) help to form bone and ossification (os-e-fik-kay-shun) hardens bone. Bone tissue resembles reinforced concrete. Collagen (call-ah-gin), threads of fibrous protein reinforce the hard cement created by calcium and phosphorus compounds.

Further, concentric rings of bone fibers called Haversian spaces (hav-er-sh-on) surround canals that contain nerve fibers and blood vessels. Osteocytes (os-t-o-sites) are cells that help maintain bone structure. During adulthood bone continually rejuvenates itself by breaking down and rebuilding. Osteoclasts (os-t-o-klasts) break bone down and osteoblasts return to build new. Calcium is very important to the action of the osteoblasts.

The **Spinal Column** is also called the vertebral column. The bones in the spine are called vertebrae (ver-ta-bray). The column starts at the base of the skull and continues to the pelvis. Alternate layers of bone (vertebrae) and cartilage (car-til-ledge, the interverte-bral discs) stack vertically one on top of the other in the spinal column. The lattice-like structure of the cancellous bone (cancel-lus, the spongy interior) in a vertebra absorbs external pressure.

The cartilaginous discs between vertebrae absorb and distribute shock and keep the vertebrae from grinding together during movement. See Figure 1, Page 144.

The spine has four natural curves. Two are lordotic (lor-dot-ick) and two are kyphotic (kye-fah-tick). The cervical and lumbar curves are lordotic. The thoracic (thor-as-ick) and sacral (say-kral) curves are kyphotic. The curves help to distribute mechanical stress as the body moves.

A **Vertebra** (ver-ta-bra) is one spinal segment or level. The term vertebrae refers to more than one spinal segment or level. The atlas, axis, cervical spine, tho-racic spine, lumbar spine (lum-bar), sacrum (say-krum), and coccyx (cock-six) are the bony elements of the spinal column.

The **Atlas and Axis** are the first two cervical (sir-ve-kal) vertebrae below the skull. These structures do not look like typical vertebrae. The atlas is ring shaped. It balances and supports the head. The axis has a tooth-like projection (called the odontoid process, oh-don-toyed) that fits up into the atlas. The combination of these two structures allows the head to turn from side to side. The atlas pivots around the axis. See Figure 2, Page 145.

Five **Cervical** vertebrae follow below the atlas and axis. The **Thoracic** spine is located in the chest area and contains 12 vertebrae. The ribs connect to the thoracic spine and protect many vital organs. Next is the **Lumbar** spine. Most people have five lumbar vertebrae although it is not unusual to have six. The lumbar vertebrae are larger than the cervical or thoracic as this spinal region carries most of the body's weight. The sacrum and coccyx are uniquely shaped.

Medical professionals often abbreviate the levels (vertebrae) of the spinal column. For example, the seven cervical vertebrae are C1, C2, C3, C4, C5, C6 and C7. The thoracic levels are T1, T2, and T3 through T12. Similarly the lumbar levels are L1 through L5 (or L6). The sacrum is simply S1. The coccyx is not abbreviated or numbered. With the exception of the atlas, axis, **Sacrum** and **Coccyx**, each cervical, thoracic, and lumbar vertebra is similarly shaped. Figure 3, Page 146, illustrates the individual components of one vertebral segment.

Intervertebral Discs separate each vertebra. A disc is made of fibrocartilage (fybro-car-til-ledge). Fibrocartilage is a type of cartilage consisting of a dense matrix of collagen fibers giving discs great tensile strength.

Discs function to absorb and distribute shock from movement (e.g. walking) and prevent the vertebrae from grinding against one another. See Figure 4, Page 147.

A disc is similar to a donut with jelly filling. The outer donut part is called the anulus fibrosus (an-you-lus fye-bro-sis) and the inner filling is the nucleus pulposus (nu-klee-us pul-poe-sis). The term "anulus" is also correctly spelled "annulus". The anulus fibrosus is made up of strong circular layers of fibrocartilage that encase the nucleus pulposus, an elastic gel-like substance. Endplates hold each intervertebral disc between the upper and lower vertebrae.

Facet Joints (fah-set) are also called **Zygapophyseal Joints** (zye-gap-o-fiz-e-al). These joints are located in the posterior spine and help to enable spinal movement. The cervical, thoracic and lumbar vertebrae each have a pair of facet joints. The facets from the upper and lower vertebrae join together (like entwined fingers) to form a facet joint. Like other joints in the body, the articulating surfaces (ar-tick-you-late-ing) are coated with smooth cartilage to facilitate movement. See Figure 5, Page 148.

The **Spinal Cord, Nerve Roots**, and the brain make up the Central Nervous System (CNS). The spinal cord is about 18 inches long; three quarter's of an inch thick and is flexible. It is the core of the communication system between the brain and the body.

The spinal bones, cerebrospinal fluid (sir-ee-bro-spinal), and three membranes called meninges (men-in-jez) protect the spinal cord. The spinal cord runs through a hollow canal created by the vertebral arches (ver-tee-brawl).

The three membranes are called the dura mater (doo-rah-matter), arachnoid membrane (ah-rack-noid), and the pia mater (pee-ah matter). The dura mater is a tough outer layer and the arachnoid is a web-like membrane that attaches to the pia mater (thin membrane closest to the spinal cord). See Figure 6, Page 149.

Thirty-one pairs of spinal nerve root fibers pass through the vertebral foramen (foe-ray-men). Similar to tree branches, nerve roots outside the spinal canal branch out to form thousands of nerve pathways throughout the body. The nerves beyond the spinal nerve roots make up the Peripheral Nervous System (PNS). Dermatomes (dur-ma-tomes) are part of the PNS. These are nerve roots that innervate the skin. See Figure 7, Page 150.

The spinal cord ends near the first lumbar vertebra (L1). From that point the nerves resemble the tail of a horse and is therefore called the cauda equina (caw-dah e-kwhy-nah).

Ligaments (lig-ah-ments) connect bone to bone and **Tendons** (ten-duns) attach muscle to bone. Ligaments and tendons are fibrous connective tissues made up of densely packed collagen fibers. Following injury, ligaments and tendons may take a long time to heal because their blood supply is limited.

In the spine, ligaments help to provide structural stability. There are two primary ligament systems in the spine, the intrasegmental and intersegmental systems. The intrasegmental system holds individual vertebrae together. The intrasegmental system includes the ligamentum flavum (lig-ah-men-tum flay-vum), interspinous (inter-spy-nus) and intertransverse (inter-tranz-verse) ligaments. The intersegmental system holds many vertebrae together.

The intersegmental system includes the anterior and posterior longitudinal ligaments, and the supraspinous (sue-pra-spine-us) ligaments. See Figure 8, Page 151.

More than 30 **Muscles** and tendons help to provide spinal balance, stability, and mobility. Usually working in groups, muscles contract and relax in response to nerve impulses that originate in the brain. Nerve impulses travel from the brain through the spinal cord to a specific location in the body via the peripheral nervous system.

There are different types of vertebral muscle; forward flexors, lateral flexors, rotators, and extensors. Muscle is the only type of body tissue with the ability to contract. It becomes shorter and thicker during contraction. Some muscles work in pairs or as antagonists. This means when a muscle contracts the opposing muscle relaxes. Muscles, tendons, and ligaments support the spine, hold it upright and control movement during rest and activity.

Several layers of fibrous connective tissue called fascia (fay-sha) cover muscles. Fascia extends beyond the muscle to become the tendon that attaches the muscle to bone.

The spinal column's **Blood Supply** (vascular system) is an elaborate system of arteries and veins. Circulation nourishes the cells in the vertebrae, spinal cord, nerves, muscles, and other structures.

Cells need plasma to reproduce and repair damage. Red blood carries oxygen to cells (e.g. muscle) to burn glucose for energy. White blood cells help fight infection and are important for immunity. A healthy vascular system helps the spine to fight disease and heal injuries.

Conclusion

It is not necessary to know the names of individual nerves and muscles, nor do you need to know how complex chemical changes in blood affect muscle contraction.

What is important is to be able to identify basic spinal elements to help understand a spinal disorder. In the chapters that follow, you will learn about spinal disorders and how they are diagnosed and treated.

Chapter 3

Consulting a Spine Specialist

Eighty percent (80%) of the population will experience neck or back pain at some point during their life. For some patients a spine disorder is a one-time inconvenience. Other patients suffer episodic pain throughout life. Pain may be accompanied by neurological sensations such as numbness and tingling in the arms or legs. It should not surprise you to learn that back pain is the number one reason people seek medical attention. Some people first visit their primary care physician. Fortunately, most disorders are not as serious as they are painful. For example, sprains and strains are very common and are easily treated. Other disorders may require the expertise of a spine specialist.

What is a spine specialist?
Spine specialists are physicians who have completed additional years of medical training to diagnose and treat disorders effecting spine. These disorders include scoliosis (sko-lee-oh-sis), osteoarthritis (os-t-o-arth-rye-tis), osteoporosis (os-t-o-pour-o-sis), herniated discs (her-knee-ate-ed), spinal stenosis (spinal sten-oh-sis), traumatic injury, fractured vertebra (ver-ta-bra), spinal deformity, tumors, infection of the spine, and congenital abnormalities. Orthopaedic Spine Surgeons and Neurosurgeons may be fellowship-trained specialists in this field. The primary care physician may provide a referral to a spine specialist.

How do I prepare for the appointment?
Consulting a spine specialist is similar to a visit with your primary care physician except the focus is on the spine. The consultation includes a physical and neurological examination during which time your medical history and symptoms are discussed. It is important

to be able to effectively communicate with the physician. The following suggestions may help you to be better prepared:

- Write down your medical history, family history, and all medications including over-the-counter drugs, vitamins, and herbs. Include allergies and side effects experienced from medications taken in the past.

- Make a list of your symptoms. Describe the type of pain, location, when it started and activities that aggravate your symptoms.

- If you recently had diagnostic testing such as an x-ray or blood work, bring a copy of the report(s). If possible, bring the actual x-ray, MRI, CT Scan, or other imaging studies performed.

- Bring the names and telephone numbers of other medical professionals who are currently treating you or have treated you for this condition in the past.

- Make a list of all your questions and concerns.

- Some patients have found it beneficial to bring a family member or friend.

What should I expect at the specialist's office?
You will be asked to complete forms to provide information about your medical and family history, previous surgery(ies), allergies, and current medications.

Many spine specialists use a universal pain diagram, which you may be asked to complete. The diagram illustrates the front and back of the body. The patient indicates where pain is felt, its intensity, the type of pain (e.g. stabbing), and other sensations such as numbness or pins and needles.

Before you meet with the physician, a medical assistant may weigh you, measure your height, and take your blood pressure and temperature. When you meet with the physician he (or she) will review the written information you have provided. The physician will ask when the symptoms began, if the onset of symptoms was sudden or gradual, if pain radiates into the extremities (e.g. arms, legs) and what event preceded the pain and/or other symptoms (e.g. motor vehicle accident). Further, the physician will want to know how your current condition affects your life. Is the condition preventing you from driving, working, or other activities of daily living (e.g. walking)?

What happens during the Physical Examination?
You will be asked to change into a gown to allow the physician to inspect the spine. During the exam your shoulders and hips are checked to determine if they are of equal height bilaterally (left, right sides). Your range of motion is observed while turning your head from side to side, bending your head to the side ear to shoulder, bending forward at the waist to touch your toes, bending at the waist to the side and then backward, and twisting your shoulders from side to side.

Next the physician may inspect and palpate (feel) your spine for muscle tenderness and spasm. While supine (lying) the physician may perform straight leg raises. Straight leg testing may be combined while you dorsiflex each foot. This means the toes are pointed toward the head. Leg length is measured using a tape measure.

What happens during the Neurological Examination?
The extent of the motor and sensory evaluation may be dependent on your symptoms and the outcome of the physical examination. A typical neurological examination may include the following:

•You may be asked to walk across the room and back, walk heel-to-toe, walk on your toes, and walk on your heels. During this time, the physician observes your posture, balance, and arms and legs during movement.

•Stand with both feet together without arm support while the physician observes the your balance. This test is repeated with the eyes open and then closed. This is called the Romberg Test.

•The physician provides resistance as you actively move to resist the force. For example, while sitting, you may be asked to lift your left knee and hold it while the physician gently tries to push the knee downward. Resistance exercises test muscle strength, flexion, and extension.

•Your ability to perceive sensation bilaterally (left and right sides) may be tested using a pinwheel instrument. For example, to test leg sensation, the physician may gently roll a pinwheel up and down the outside of each calf. You will be asked if the sensation is felt equally in both the left and right calves. A tuning fork tests your ability to perceive vibration.

•Reflexes are tested using a rubber tipped reflex hammer. The hammer is gently tapped against one or more tendons in your arms and legs. Reflexes may be tested while you are sitting or lying down.

•Eye movement is observed as you watch the physician's finger move left to right, up and down.

Conclusion
The information obtained from both examinations help to form the diagnosis. Diagnostic tests confirm the diagnosis. To learn about diagnostic testing, read the following chapter.

Chapter 4

Diagnostic Tests

Fred has come to see his physician today because he has a backache. The conversation between Fred and his physician went something like this -- "Well Fred, when did the pain start?" - Fred replies, "Oh a couple of hours after I played a game of golf." - Physician, "How many holes did you play?" - Fred responds, "36 – it was a great day for golf!" The physician asks when Fred last played golf, to which Fred responds, "Oh, about six months ago."

After the physician and Fred talk a little longer and following an examination, it appears the condition is not serious. It is back sprain or strain, a soft tissue problem. In this case, Fred's backache did not even require even an x-ray.

Of course not all back and neck problems are so easy to diagnose. Some spinal disorders require an x-ray, CT Scan, or MRI. Diagnostic tools have rapidly advanced along with other technologies. It is not uncommon for a patient to ask about a specific test. The following information is provided to help answer some of these questions.

X-Ray is the most common test performed today. In 1895, Wilhelm Conrad Roentgen discovered the x-ray. His remarkable achievement radically changed the practice of medicine. For the first time physicians could see beyond the skin and underlying soft tissues to the skeleton without autopsy. Roentgen did not entirely understand these unusual rays. He used the letter "x" to describe the rays because in Algebra "x" refers to an unknown.

When the spine is x-rayed the beams pass through the skin and underlying soft tissues (e.g. muscle, ligaments, tendons). When the beams meet bone (vertebra) it stops creating a white shadow on the film. A bone abnormality is reflected on the finished film. Shades of gray mirror the density of the different tissues. X-rays are best for looking at bone. They are not helpful for looking at soft trauma.

X-rays are widely used today and are often called radiographs. These tests are not performed at random. An x-ray would most likely be performed when spine or extremity pain (e.g. leg, arm) is severe or chronic and progressive. An x-ray may rule out particular problems involving bone and some soft tissue disorders. When an x-ray proves inconclusive additional tests may be ordered especially if something suspicious is detected.

CT Scan (Computerized Axial Tomography) or CAT Scan was developed in 1970. The CT Scan evolved from Tomograms; multiple x-rays taken at different levels to check the depth of an abnormality. The advent of computers in medicine has meant less radiation exposure and shorter study times. The CT Scan has become an important adjunct to x-rays. The CT Scan uses multiple x-ray beams projected at many angles in conjunction with computer resources to create three-dimensional cross-sectional images. Each image or picture reveals a different level of tissue that resembles slices.

MRI (Magnetic Resonance Imaging) is one of the most sensitive diagnostic tools. This medical miracle was first used on humans in 1971.

MRIs differ from CT Scans in that there is no exposure to radiation. The MRI equipment is basically two powerful magnets; one external and one internal. Within the human body there are millions of negative and positive charged atoms. When these atoms are exposed to the electromagnetic waves produced by the MRI equipment, the atoms act like mini-magnets. By means of a computer, the data is collected, combined, and manipulated using complex mathematical equations. The final product reveals detailed anatomical images transferred onto film. MRI represents the gold standard in imaging. MRI is best for looking at soft tissues such as discs or nerves.

To appreciate the details rendered by an MRI consider the following contrast. Under x-ray, an intervertebral disc resembles a pocket of air. Using MRI the structure of the same disc is revealed in fine detail. Additionally, contrast dye introduced into the patient intravenously further defines and highlights particular aspects of the spine.

There are a few drawbacks to MRI. For example, take 100 normal people who appear to have nothing wrong with their spines and perform an MRI on each. The results may reveal that 20-25% of asymptomatic participants (without symptoms) have a herniated or bulging disc, or an arthritic condition. These patients are pain free and their lives go on without interruption at that particular time. The disadvantage is the results of an MRI may create a false positive. This means the MRI revealed a disorder for which there are no corresponding clinical symptoms. The point is this - the clinical symptoms must coincide with test results. It is not uncommon for a patient to come to the physician with a stack of MRIs indicating a herniated disc.

Lets say the patient is a competitive tennis player without clinical symptoms indicative of a herniated disc. In this case, to give the patient a serious diagnosis based simply on an MRI would be inappropriate. This is why MRI results must support the patient's clinical symptoms for a specific disorder. In some cases, a bulging disc does not cause any pain or problem. If leg pain is present and the MRI indicates a herniated disc associated with the nerves to the leg, it confirms the herniation as the cause of the leg pain.

For patients who are claustrophobic (claw-stro-foe-bick, fear of confinement) open-air MRI equipment is available. These patient-friendly imaging tables produce an excellent image without confinement in an imaging tube. Medicine to relax the patient is available and can be administered prior to the test.

Patients with internal ferromagnetic (metallic iron) devices such as a pacemaker, metal cardiac valve or metal in the area of the exam cannot be scanned. The powerful MRI magnets would interfere with these metal devices. In these patients a CT Scan is performed.

A **Bone Scan** may help to detect very fine stress fractures, arthritis, infections, or tumors. The patient is first injected with a liquid material that settles into the bone over a period of a few hours. During the test, the patient lies on the scanning table and a camera moves back and forth over the entire body.

An area of increased activity will light up brighter (termed a hot spot or spot) than other parts possibly indicating a problem. This is a nonspecific test. When the results are positive (meaning abnormal) further investigation may be needed.

Bone Density Scan is also called a **Bone Mineral Density (BMD)** test. This test measures the density or compactness of bone and is important in the diagnosis of osteoporosis (os-t-o-pour-o-sis).

Further, a bone density scan may provide an early warning for the risk of developing osteoporosis. Computerized scanning equipment using a low dose of radiation measures bone density in the hip and spine. The test takes about 15 minutes.

Nerve Function Tests
Electromyography (elec-tro-my-ah-gra-fee, EMG), Nerve Conduction Velocity (NCV) and Discography (dis-ah-gra-fee) are tests used to confirm or deny nerve involvement.

Sciatica (sy-attic-ka) is a symptom presenting as pain that radiates from the buttock down the leg. Nerve tests help to answer the question "is the pain coming from a leg muscle or is it a sign of nerve compression in the spine?"

Electromyography (EMG) may be used to determine if muscle function is normal or abnormal. An EMG tests for the nerve impulse coming from the brain and spinal cord. The nerve pulse is followed enroute to its final destination to determine if the nerve is blocked or delayed and where.

Nerve Conduction Velocity (NCV) is a sensitive test that is performed with an EMG. NCV stimulates a specific nerve and records the nerve's ability to transmit an impulse. This study may reveal where the nerve is unable to function normally.

Discography or a discogram is a type of x-ray used to view the intervertebral disc space. The abnormal disc is injected with an illuminating fluid under x-ray. The fluid injection may replicate the patient's symptoms, which may include leg pain. Abnormalities related to disc function or anatomical disorders might be determined by discography.

Laboratory Tests

A simple blood test may reveal infection, tumor or other spinal condition. Sometimes these disorders cannot be seen on an x-ray.

A urinalysis (yu-ri-nal-is-sis) may reveal kidney stones or infection, which may cause severe back pain. Further, a urinalysis may detect by-products from muscle breakdown created by trauma or muscle disease.

In Summary

Osteoporosis (os-t-o-pour-o-sis) is an excellent example how diagnostic tests are used to help prevent and diagnose disease. When osteoporosis is found early, it can be easily treated.

To learn about other spinal disorders, refer to the following chapter, Common Spinal Disorders.

Chapter 5

Common Spinal Disorders

There are many types of back and neck disorders that affect the majority of the population in the United States. Injury, aging, general health, and lifestyle may influence the development of some conditions. Most spinal disorders are known to result from soft tissue injury, structural injury, and degenerative, or congenital conditions.

Soft Tissue Injuries

Soft tissues include the muscles, tendons (ten-duns), ligaments (lig-ah-ments), and nerves. Injury to these tissues can be caused by unnecessary stress to the spine. To give you an idea of how stress affects the spine, consider the following information. Keep in mind the numbers are relatively accurate when proper posture and body mechanics are used.

Lying flat on the back, very little pressure is exerted on the spine. As a person stands upright the pressure climbs *three* times and while sitting *four* times. Forces affecting the lower back can rise *five* times as a medium weight box is lifted. But what happens when poor posture is combined with faulty body mechanics? Those numbers would escalate as the following example demonstrates:

Poor Body Mechanics: Bending at the waist instead of at the knees to pick something lightweight up off the floor. This movement may cause as much as *10 times* the amount of unnecessary stress to the spine. Micro-trauma or mini-injuries to soft tissue may result from improper movement especially when repetitive. It is not surprising why so many people suffer from back and neck pain.

39

Sprains and Strains affect soft tissue. By definition both conditions mean something has stretched beyond normal. Consider Dave who has not shoveled snow since last winter and has decided to take care of his driveway after the first big storm. More than likely Dave's back and neck muscles will become strained causing pain, tenderness, and stiffness. Why? Dave forced his muscles to perform beyond what he does on a routine basis.

Muscle tissue may become strained when forced to exceed its ability to work. Regular exercise helps to strengthen muscles, allowing them to work harder longer. Muscles are the spine's workhorses. Besides muscle tissue, sprains and strains can affect a ligament or tendon. Ligaments attach bone to bone and tendons attach muscle to bone. A sprained ankle is an example of a sprained ligament.

The bulk of the back is muscle. Extreme force may injure muscle. During a motor vehicle accident the body may be suddenly thrown forward, backward, and sideways. These movements can cause hyperextension (excessive forward movement) and hyperflexion (excessive backward movement), which can cause muscles, ligaments, and tendons to tear.

The symptoms of sprain and strain include sudden, sharp, and persistent pain at the injury site followed by swelling. The patient may think a bone has broken.

If medical attention is sought, the physician will ask several questions about the injury during the physical examination. When indicated, an x-ray is performed to rule out abnormality (e.g. broken bone). The physician may prescribe medication to treat pain, inflammation, and spasm during the healing phase.

Following injury, the soft tissues switch into high gear to begin the healing process. Circulating blood quickly carries nutrition to the injury and carries away waste. Sprains and strains are usually self-healing within a two to three week time period.

Treatment may include physical therapy accompanied by a stretching program to help prevent the formation of scar tissue, which can be debilitating. Scar tissue is not normal tissue but is the result of healing. Consider scars that develop on the skin after a severe burn. In most cases the scars are with the patient for life, unless surgically removed. In the case of muscles, ligaments, and tendons a physical therapist may be able to train the scar tissue to mimic the function of the tissue prior to injury. Where a ligament has torn scar tissue can be used to aid in providing some limited strength.

Muscle Spasms are common. Muscles that have not been conditioned may not be able to handle added demands. When a muscle is overworked or overstretched its response is to go into spasm. The pain produced by muscle spasm can be so severe the patient is fearful that something serious is wrong. The intensity of the pain can be disabling and affect posture (e.g. bent to one side).

Whiplash is a hyperextension and hyperflexion injury that may cause micro-trauma to the soft tissues in the neck and upper back. The forces to the spine incurred during a car accident may cause the head and neck to suddenly and rapidly move forward, backward, and side ways. Muscles, ligaments, and tendons in the spine may become stretched beyond normal limits causing micro-trauma or small tears in the muscles, ligaments, and tendons. Symptoms may include pain, burning sensations, and headache.

Treatment for whiplash may include a soft cervical collar to help lift some of the skull's weight off tender neck, shoulder and back tissues. The collar helps to immobilize and protect the cervical area during the initial healing stage. In most cases, whiplash is self-limiting. It heals over a four to six week time period. Sometimes whiplash may cause long lasting (chronic) problems of a nonsurgical nature. Rarely does whiplash create a severe disorder requiring surgery.

Spinal Nerve Disorders

Compressive Neuropathy (nu-rop-ah-thee) occurs when nerves in the spine are compressed. This disorder often affects older people. The nerves that exit the spinal canal become trapped, compressed, and swollen. Foraminal stenosis can be extremely painful and debilitating. The effects may temporarily damage or permanently destroy nerves. Foraminal stenosis (foe-ray-min-al sten-oh-sis, e.g. spinal stenosis) is an example of a compressive neuropathy.

A slipped, herniated (her-knee-ate-ed), ruptured or bulging disc may cause nerve compression. Nerves may also be compressed or even displaced by the growth of bone spurs. A compressive neuropathy may cause pain to radiate into one or both buttocks, down the legs below the knees and may be felt in the ankles and feet. Pain may be accompanied by sensations of tingling, numbness, and weakness. These types of symptoms are generally referred to as "sciatica."

Sciatica (sy-attic-ka) is a symptom of a compressive neuropathy involving one or several of the lower spinal nerves that make up the sciatic nerve. It is a common ailment named for the sciatic nerve, which is a collection of smaller nerves descending from the spine and joining together to resemble a cable. The spinal nerves come together in the pelvis to form the sciatic nerve.

42

The sciatic nerve then travels down through each buttock into the legs. At certain points, such as in the posterior thighs, nerves branch off from the main sciatic cable. This is why sciatic pain may be felt in various muscles of the leg. See Figure 9, Page 152.

A direct blow to the sciatic nerve in the leg may occur when falling down. This may injure the sciatic nerve. The force from falling down could initiate bleeding around the nerve and cause nerve compression and pain. If a disc or bone spur protrudes into the spinal nerves that become the sciatic nerve, the problem may become severe. A bone spur could displace a spinal nerve creating intense pain. Fortunately there are non-surgical treatments available to help reduce inflammation and associated pain. These treatments include medication and steroid injections.

When nonsurgical treatment fails and, depending on the patient's symptomatology, surgery may be considered. In some cases a surgical procedure called a laminotomy (lamb-in-ah-toe-me) may be performed to give the surgeon greater access to the offending intervertebral disc. Removal of the disc is called a discectomy or microdiscectomy (under magnification).

Peripheral Neuropathy is a degenerative, toxic, or nutritional condition affecting the nerves that branch into the body's extremities such as the arms, hands, legs, and feet. Diabetes or even certain drugs can cause peripheral neuropathy. The disease causes the peripheral or distant parts of nerves to shrink. Eventually the affected nerves may deteriorate to the point that the nerves can no longer carry impulses. Sensory (feeling) and motor (movement) function may be lost. Symptoms may include burning or a feeling of pins and needles, numbness in the toes or fingers, and weakness when gripping an object or while walking. Medicacation may help to slow the effects of peripheral neuropathy but may not cure or stops its progression.

Spinal Infections are rare and painful. Immediate medical attention is always necessary. If an infection is not detected and treated, the effected area swells and causes pain to radiate into adjoining tissue. A spinal infection may cause permanent injury or take root in the epidural cavity (ep-e-do-ral). This cavity is a fatty area near nerve roots and provides space for an infection or abscess. Epidural cavities are found in the cervical (sir-ve-kal), thoracic (thor-as-ick), and lumbar (lum-bar) spine. An MRI may be performed to confirm a spinal infection. Nonsurgical treatment may include intravenous or oral antibiotics combined with bed rest. In some cases surgical intervention may be necessary to eradicate the infection.

Spinal Meningitis (men-in-ji-tis) is an infection that causes inflammation of the membranes in the brain and spinal cord. This is a serious disease and may require hospitalization. Treatment includes intravenous or oral antibiotics combined with bed rest. Symptoms may include fever, weakness, pain that radiates from the spine, muscle spasm, sensitivity to touch, decreased spinal flexibility, fatigue, sweating, and weight loss. When a child is affected, symptoms may include his refusal to stand or sit because it is painful. Increased backache may be an indication in older children and adults. Neck pain and sensitivity to light are common symptoms.

Structural Injuries
Structural injuries are those affecting the bones and discs. Nerve roots may become irritated or damaged when injury involves a vertebra (ver-ta-bra) or disc. Pain and weakness are symptoms that may accompany a structural injury.

Spinal Fractures are different from a broken arm or leg. A spinal fracture may involve the spinal cord. The spinal column is the spinal cord's suit of armor. Damage to the armor could cause injury to the spinal cord and any of its 31 pairs of nerve roots. Fractures in the spine may include the vertebral (ver-tee-brawl) body and its attachments such as the facet joints (fah-set), pars articularis (parz are-tick-you-lar-es), and spinous process. Damage to any of these bony elements may cause injury to the spinal cord and nerve structures. See Figure 10, Page 153.

Compression Fractures are the most common. The vertebral body is the largest single unit of a vertebra. Its structural integrity is similar to a cardboard box. Visualize a cardboard box. It appears to be big and sturdy but is hollow inside. Sudden and excessive force to the box creates pressure. Force can cause the box to crush into a wedge shape. The force is distributed and may affect other spinal structures.

It could be assumed that the smaller cervical (sir-ve-kal) vertebrae would be more susceptible to injury based on size. Compression fractures do not occur as often in the lumbar spine because these vertebrae are the largest and most dense.

Other fractures may result from forces that cause the body to torque (twist). Even a direct blow to the spine can cause fracture. Others parts of the vertebra including the facet joints or other bony processes may break causing vertebral dislocation and paralysis.

Although bone is a hard material it can crack, split, or break away from the parent bone. Spinal fractures require immediate medical attention. An unstable fracture can be a serious condition causing bone fragments to press against the spinal cord or nerves.

Osteoporosis (os-t-o-pour-o-sis) is a disease that adversely effects bone density. It can cause bones to become porous, weak, and sometimes delicate as porcelain. Osteoporotic bone is especially susceptible to fracture.The type of fracture is diagnosed by x-ray. Treatment depends on the type of fracture and the location. Some fractures require surgical intervention and others require bracing to stabilize the spine. The first step is to stop movement to control and minimize injury.

When a vertebra fractures the body's first response is to begin healing. Initially a granular material called a callus is formed at the fracture site. Collagen (call-ah-gin), a protein is transported to the site through the blood stream. Collagen helps to mend and knit the fracture together. After new bone is joined with the old bone it is hardened through a process called calcification (kal-see-fi-cay-shun).

Plastics have revolutionized the brace and cast business today. Years ago a patient with a broken back had no other choice than to wear a plaster cast. Today, casts and braces are made from plastics and other materials. Braces are custom-fitted, removable, and designed to be comfortable. Today, most spinal fractures are more of an inconvenience than a tragedy.

Spondylolisthesis (spon-de-low-lis-thee-sis) means one vertebra slips over the one below. This disease primarily affects the elderly as a degenerative disease but, it can be congenital (present at birth) or discovered early in life.

Childhood spondylolisthesis may result if the pars articularis (parz are-tick-you-lar-es) does not fuse during early development. Posterior vertebral weakness results when these bony elements do not grow together. Spondylolisthesis may occur following injury or overuse because the bony weakness makes the area weak and susceptible to break. A spine expert is best qualified to treat this condition.

Elderly or degenerative spondylolisthesis develops when the stabilizing spinal structures begin to deteriorate. This usually occurs in the lower back, which carries most of the body's weight. See Figure 11, Page 154.

Sometimes the spinal joints become arthritic and wear out, which may cause spinal instability. As vertebrae (ver-ta-bray) lose normal alignment one vertebra may slip forward over the vertebra below it. When this happens the neural foramina (space where nerves leave the spinal canal) may become closed causing nerve compression and sciatica. This condition is similar to spinal stenosis.

In most cases, spondylolisthesis is treated non-surgically. Treatment may include a course of physical therapy, steroid-anesthetic injections, and medication (prescription or over-the-counter) for inflammation and pain.

When nonsurgical treatment fails, and depending on the patient's symptoms, a surgical procedure may be considered. In cases of severe slippage or instability, a spinal fusion may be necessary. Spinal fusion helps to stabilize the weak area of the spine using rods, screws, or plates, and bone graft.

Leg pain, weakness, or numbness may be alleviated by a surgical procedure called a foraminotomy (for-am-not-toe-me). This procedure increases the size of the neuroforamen and cleans away debris that clogs the neural foramina.

Abnormal Spinal Curvature

Scoliosis (sko-lee-oh-sis) is a term taken from a Greek word meaning curvature. During the 19th Century physicians thought poor posture was the primary cause of scoliosis. Today scoliosis is known to be either congenital (present at birth) or developmental and may be hereditary. The disease causes the spine to curve laterally (to the side) usually in the shape of an "S" or "C". The curve is measured in degrees. Some curves are severe. See Figure 12, Page 155.

Idiopathic Scoliosis (id-dee-oh-path-ick sko-lee-oh-sis) is the childhood version of adult scoliosis. It is hereditary and primarily affects healthy young girls during their early teens. Physical signs may include uneven shoulders, one hip lower than the other, a rib hump when bent over at the waist and leaning to one side. When maturity is reached the disease may stabilize or slowly degenerate over time. In an adult with scoliosis, the curve may have begun to develop during childhood but went unnoticed.

Whatever the patient's age, the goal is to stabilize the spine to prevent additional curvature. Some patients with scoliosis are pain free and do not seek treatment until deformity is noticed. Unfortunately, at that point it may be too late to treat the disease.

The size of the curve is measured in degrees on an x-ray. The progression of scoliosis is monitored by periodic x-ray studies. When scoliosis is severe it may cause the spine to rotate, which can cause spinal spacing to narrow on the opposite side of the body.

Kyphosis (ky-foe-sis) is the normal curvature of the rib-bearing thoracic spine. Excessive kyphosis may develop as a result of poor posture early in life. Kyphosis means the spine is bent forward. Although kyphosis usually affects women, it is found to develop in men too. An excessive form of kyphosis may cause a hump to form in the shoulder blade area of the upper back. Kyphosis may affect men and women with osteoporosis. See Figure 13, Page 156.

Lordosis (lor-doe-sis) is the normal contour of the neck and lower back. Excessive lordosis may cause an extreme inward curve in the lower back. This condition is also called swayback. See Figure 14, Page 157.

Disorders Affecting Intervertebral Discs
Herniated and Bulging Discs
In lay terms, a slipped disc can mean a ruptured disc or herniated disc (her-knee-ate-ed). See Figure 15, Page 158. Although the term slipped disc is used, discs do not slip. Each intervertebral disc is sandwiched between two vertebrae supported by a system of ligaments that help hold the spinal package together.

Disc disorders are contained or non-contained. A bulging disc is an example of a contained disc disorder. A bulging disc has not broken open; the nucleus pulposus (new-klee-us pul-poe-sis) remains contained within the anulus fibrosus (an-you-lus fye-bro-sis). A bulging disc could be compared to a volcano prior to eruption and may be a precursor to herniation. The disc may protrude into the spinal canal without breaking open. The gel-like interior (nucleus pulposus) does not leak out. The disc remains intact except a small bubble pops out attached to the disc.

A non-contained disc is one that has either partially or completely broken open; a herniated or ruptured disc. To illustrate imagine a tube (anulus fibrosus) of toothpaste (nucleus pulposus) placed under pressure. The pressure causes the toothpaste within the tube to move wherever it can. If any part of the tube is weak

49

toothpaste may leak out. When a disc herniates the contents may spread out to the spinal cord and nerves. The disc material has little space to go --- into the area occupied by the spinal canal and nerve roots.

Returning to the leaky tube of toothpaste, the disc's gel-like nucleus contains a chemical that irritates the nerves causing them to swell. After the chemical agent has done its job, the remnants of the chemical remain and continue to press on the irritated and swollen nerves. To complicate matters, sometimes fragments from the anulus (tire-like outer disc wall) break away from the parent disc and drift into the spinal canal. These free fragments may travel in the spinal canal. Depending on the type of injury and the condition of the discs, more than one disc may herniate, rupture, or bulge. Sometimes injury causes a combination of disc disorders.

Degenerative and Congenital Disorders
Degenerative disorders may develop as a result of the normal aging process and wear and tear. Just like a mechanical device the human body is subject to wear and tear from use. However, unlike machinery, the human body has the ability to heal or attempt to repair itself.

At birth the structural integrity of the spine, heart, lungs, and other organ systems is at its peak for future development. During mid-life early microscopic changes begin to appear that indicate the spine is aging. The spine does not deteriorate just because of age. Wear and tear is also responsible. Disorders such as arthritis (arth-rye-tis), spinal stenosis (spinal sten-oh-sis), and osteoporosis (os-t-o-pour-o-sis) do not develop overnight. Degenerative diseases may take years to develop and may be associated with past injury, abuse, body structure, or congenital problems.

Arthritis affects approximately 80% of people over the age of 55 in the United States. Injury, a weakened immune system, and/or hereditary factors can trigger the onset of arthritis. There are hundreds of types of arthritis that share similar symptoms including inflammation, joint pain, and progressive deterioration of joint surfaces over time. The joints may lose normal contour, excessive amounts of fluid may build up inside the joint along with pieces of floating debris. Arthritis may affect the joints in the spine, which enable the body to bend and twist. Part of the problem may be the body's response to arthritis, which is to manufacture extra bone to stop joint movement. The extra bone is called a bone spur or bony overgrowth. See Figure 15, 158.

In medical terms, the extra bone is called an osteophyte (os-t-o-fight). Osteophytes may be found in areas affected by arthritis such as the disc or joint spaces where cartilage has deteriorated. The body's production of osteophytes is a futile attempt to stop the motion of the arthritic joint and deal with the degenerative process. It never completely works. The evidence of bony deposits can be found on an x-ray.

A bone spur may cause nerve impingement at the neuroforamen (nu-row for-a-men). The neuroforamen are passageways through which the nerve roots exit the spinal canal. Sensory symptoms include pain, numbness, burning and pins and needles in the extremities below the affected spinal nerve root. Motor symptoms include muscle spasm, cramping, weakness, or loss of muscular control in a part of the body.

Osteoarthritis (OA) (os-t-o-arth-rye-tis) is the degenerative form of arthritis. It is a progressive joint disease associated with aging. Many elderly people have some degree of osteoarthritis. It may be found in the knees, hips, or other joints. Spinal osteoarthritis affects the facet joints that enable the body to bend and twist. As the facet joints deteriorate, cartilage may become inflamed and start to fray like a well-used rag. During this process cartilage (car-til-ledge) breaks away from the joint surfaces. Cartilage fragments may begin to float in the fluid that lubricates the joint. Joints stripped of their cartilage are no longer smooth slick surfaces that enable friction-free movement. Joint bones begin to rub together while trying to work. The nerve structures in the joint become irritated and cause inflammation and pain.

Osteoarthritis may trigger the formation of osteophytes. As previously mentioned, these bony spurs are the body's way of dealing with the disease. In the spine, osteophytes may cause disc space to narrow. When this happens the affected intervertebral disc may collapse.

Rheumatoid Arthritis (RA) (room-ah-toyed arth-rye-tis) is a progressive form of arthritis that can be painfully destructive. RA may cause the interior joint tissues to swell and thicken. Over time the affected joint disintegrates leading to deformity. RA may appear during early middle age and is more common in women than men. The symptoms include fatigue, weakness, and loss of appetite, fever, and anemia. Upon rising joints are usually stiff, swollen, and tender. Medication is available to help relieve pain and inflammation. Regular exercise helps joints to function. Passive forms of physical therapy may help to increase joint mobility.

Ankylosing Spondylitis (an-key-low-sing spon-dee-lie-tis) is a chronic and progressive inflammatory disease of the spine. It is characterized by early sacroiliac joint (say-kro-ill-e-ak, sacrum) involvement followed by hardening of the anulus fibrosus and surrounding connective tissue along with arthritic changes in the facet joints. The disease may cause the spine to gradually lose flexibility and stiffen. The disease is hereditary.

Spinal Stenosis (spinal sten-oh-sis) Translated from the Greek language, stenosis means a narrowing of a normally larger opening, the spinal canal or neuroforamen (nu-row for-a-men, window) through which nerves exit the spinal column. This disorder is associated with aging. Some people are predisposed to spinal stenosis genetically or it may be caused by a congenital condition.

If the neuroforamen are partially or completely closed, the spinal nerves become compressed or trapped. The symptoms of spinal stenosis include numbness, weakness, and sensations of burning, tingling, and pins and needles in the affected extremity such as the leg. See Figure 16, Page 159.

Spinal stenosis could be compared to wearing a pair of shoes that are a half size too small. The feet (nerves) react to the pressure by swelling (inflammation) that makes the shoes even tighter. The pain (nerve compression) can make walking difficult or impossible. Patients with spinal stenosis have found the pain eases when bending forward or sitting. Bending forward creates more space between the vertebrae that may temporarily relieve nerve compression.

Spinal stenosis may affect any part of the spine but is more prevalent in the lumbar spine. Lumbar spinal stenosis produces pain that may be felt in the buttocks, thighs, and calves when walking or standing. Cervical spinal stenosis affects the upper extremities and back. When severe, cervical spinal stenosis may affect the body from the neck down.

A CT Scan or MRI is performed to confirm that the patient's symptoms are caused by spinal stenosis. When necessary a surgical procedure called a foraminotomy (for-am-not-toe-me) is performed to enlarge the size of the window to help relieve nerve compression.

Foraminal Stenosis (foe-ray-min-al sten-oh-sis) is similar to spinal stenosis but is singled out because it primarily affects one or more vertebral foramen. In a normal spine nerve roots have enough room to slip through the foramen. However, age and disease may affect the foramen by clogging the openings with debris that trap and compress nerves.

The symptoms of foraminal stenosis include numbness, weakness, and sensations of burning, tingling, and pins and needles in the affected extremity (e.g. leg). Not every stenosis is critical but if ignored nerves may die that may cause a loss of function. Functional loss may involve the ability to feel (sensory) and move (motor).

If nonsurgical treatments are unsuccessful in relieving the patient's symptoms, surgery may become an option. The procedure is called a foraminotomy and is discussed in Chapter 9, Page 76.

Degenerative Disc Disease (DDD) affects the vertebral discs. During spinal flexion and extension, the discs absorb and distribute pressure and excessive stress created by movement. It is natural for some disc wear and tear to occur with age and movement.

When the spine is x-rayed the disc spaces between the vertebrae may appear narrow indicating DDD. Loss of disc hydration is one of many biochemical changes that occurs with age and may cause discs to thin, shrink, or collapse. A similar chemical change occurs as a tire ages. As the tire loses its resilience its original form is compromised. The disc may shrink in size, wrinkle, or crack. Pieces of the disc may break away (fragments) and cause nerve irritation. Thin, collapsed, or broken discs reduce the size of the neuroforamen formed between the upper and lower vertebral discs. As the neuroforamen is reduced in size, compressed nerves begin to swell and signal pain. See Figure 15, Page 158.

The neuroforamen could be compared to brakes on a car. In this scenario the vertebral discs are the brake pads that form a cushion between the foot pedal (top vertebral body) and the wheel (bottom vertebral body). Age, abuse, and wear and tear cause the brake pads to thin or even disintegrate. What happens? The brakes squeal (pain) and may not stop the car. The driver of the car feels the affects of the faulty brakes. A   normal amount of wear and tear is expected and acceptable. The same is true of the spine. With proper nutrition, regular exercise, and prevention the body can be in good shape at any age.

Osteoporosis (os-t-o-pour-o-sis) is known as the silent degenerative disease. It is labeled silent because in the early stage of the disease the patient may be free of symptoms. However, as the disease progresses, bones gradually begin to resemble a well-used sponge, thin and porous. Bone mass and density (strength) is lost. See Figure 17, Page 160. Although spinal osteoporosis is more common, osteoporosis can affect any bone in the body. It makes bones susceptible to fracture. It could be said that osteoporosis begins when the body makes more calcium withdrawals than deposits resulting in bankrupt bones.

The symptoms of spinal osteoporosis include chronic pain, loss of mobility, and an alternation in appearance. Patients may look frail, bent over and shorter. Chronic pain may result from spinal muscles forced to handle the spine's load. Daily chores like making the bed, removing food from the oven, or even embracing a loved one can cause vertebrae (ver-ta-bray) to break.

Deformities may develop as the bones in the spine become more porous and weaker. Bone breakdown may eventually lead to compression and crush fractures as well as a hump back (excessive kyphosis). Loss of bone strength may cause spontaneous fracture. The patient's body weight alone may cause vertebrae to collapse leading to compressed nerves. As vertebrae collapse the patient loses height. Internal organs may be forced out of their normal position. Osteoporosis can be an insidious disease eventually causing health to deteriorate.

Osteoporosis is a normal part of aging for women and men. It is important to know the risk factors and reduce them. Smoking, alcoholism, heavy use of laxatives, stress, diabetes, menopause, inactivity, and unhealthy dieting are factors known to accelerate the progression of the disease. Women who smoke produce lower levels of estrogen. Plus smoking interferes with calcium absorption necessary for strong healthy bones. Alcoholics, women or men, usually have less bone mass because calcium absorption is hindered. Stress can be an undermining factor because it may stimulate adrenal hormone production that could cause calcium to be passed during urination.

Women are prone to osteoporosis because their bones are smaller and contain less mass than a man's bones. Additionally, during menopause estrogen levels are affected. Estrogen helps to maintain sufficient calcium in the skeletal system. Further, women usually live longer than men therefore, women have more time to develop osteoporosis.

A Bone Mineral Density (BMD) test is a simple, painless, and quick noninvasive test for osteoporosis. This test measures the density of bone. If signs of osteoporosis are found the physician may prescribe medication to help control the disease. Since it can take years for bone to gain strength, treatment may be started when the patient is in their 60s. The medication is available in several forms; pill, nasal spray, or transdermal patch. In some cases the medication helps to prevent spontaneous fractures or a broken hip or rib from a minor fall.

Regular exercise is especially important at any age for many reasons. Physical activity stimulates bone to become denser, increases circulation that nourishes bone, and helps to maintain healthy hormone levels. Weight bearing and resistance exercises such as walking build strong bones. Before starting any exercise program, see your physician.

Spinal Tumors are rare. The physician is interested in determining the cause of the tumor, if there is a past history of cancer, and relieving associated pain. If the patient's primary condition is breast or lung cancer it is possible for the cancer to metastasize (spread) to the spine. Tumors can occur in anyone without a history of disease. Fortunately not all spinal tumors are malignant (cancerous).

Conclusion
To learn how certain degenerative disorders affect the spine and are treated, see Chapter 10 on page 81 and Chapter 11 on page 103.

Chapter 6

Pain Management Techniques to Help Conquer Back and Neck Pain

Steven H. Richeimer, M.D.

Back and neck pain is one of the leading causes of lost work time, second only to the common cold. It affects 65-85% of the population of the United States at some point in their lives.

The most common cause is a sprain, strain, or spasm usually brought on by poor lifting techniques, improper posture, or an unhealthy ergonomic environment. Another common cause is disc problems brought on by injury, wear and tear, or age. Other causes include spinal stenosis, osteoarthritis, osteoporosis, and other conditions discussed in this book and at *spineuniverse.com*.

Pain management often takes a 'multidisciplinary approach' to minimize or eliminate pain. The goals include increasing physical activity, eliminating unsafe medication use, and learning lifestyle behaviors that work toward wellness.

The purpose of this chapter is to help you understand pain management. Included is an explanation of the different types of pain and treatments pain management specialists use to fight pain.

Types of Back and Neck Pain

Acute Pain (ah-cute pain) can be defined as severe short-term pain. Post-operative pain is an example. Acute pain is self-limiting, which means the pain acts to warn you to cease or limit activity that could cause additional tissue damage.

The more intense and prolonged an acute pain episode is, the more likely it will lead to chronic pain. This makes sense given the information that we are beginning to learn about how the central nervous system changes in response to intense pain. As a result of intense pain, neurons in the spinal cord that help to prevent pain transmissions actually die. At the same time, pain-transmitting neurons grow more connections to other nerves, become more sensitive, and react more strongly to painful stimulus.

The study of neuroplasticity (nu-row-plas-te-city, how the nervous system changes and molds itself) is one of the hottest new areas in neuroscience since it seems to be the basis for the processes of learning and memory. It appears, however, that the nervous system not only learns useful information, but also "learns" or remembers pain, leading to the development of chronic pain.

Chronic Pain. Rather than being the symptom of a disease process, chronic pain is itself a disease process. Chronic pain is unrelenting and not self-limiting. It can persist for years and even decades after the initial injury. There are many factors that affect the development of chronic pain such as age, level of disability, depression, or the presence of nerve damage.

Neuropathic Pain (nu-row-path-ick pain) is usually described by patients as burning, electric, tingling, and shooting in nature. Often, this type of pain cannot be controlled using traditional pain killing oral drugs.

Management of neuropathic pain may include other medications (that are often not thought of as pain medicines) and multiple treatment modalities such as physical therapy, physical rehabilitation, relaxation training, trigger point injections, epidural steroid injections,

Sympathetic blocks, spinal cord stimulators, intrathecal morphine pump systems, and various surgical techniques.

Nociceptive Pain (no-si-sep-tiv pain) is localized pain, which is usually described by patients as sharp, aching, or throbbing. Post-operative pain, pain associated with trauma, and arthritic pain are examples of nociceptive pain. Nociceptive pain usually responds to nonsteroidal anti-inflammatory drugs (NSAIDs) and opioids (oh-pe-oids, strong prescription pain killers).

Pain Management Treatments and Therapies
Anti-Depressant Medications

There is considerable evidence that tricyclic anti-depressants are effective for the treatment of a variety of pain conditions, such as migraine headaches and neuropathic pain.

Nonsteroidal Anti-Inflammatory Drugs (NSAIDs) are valuable analgesics (pain relieving medication). These drugs do not alter the patient's cognitive functions, cause respiratory depression, or nausea. However, NSAIDs are associated with significant side effects especially with long-term use.

Epidural Steroid Injections (ESI). The traditional epidural (ep-e-do-ral) steroid injection technique involves the physician feeling the patient's spine in order to guide the placement of a needle between the spinal vertebrae. A newer technique involves using x-ray fluoroscopy (floor-o-sko-pee) to guide the needle directly to the neural foramen, the point where the affected spinal nerve root exits the spine.

Injections of steroids into the lumbar epidural space are particularly useful for pain that radiates from the lower back into a leg. This pain may be caused by disc herniation or spinal stenosis, which triggers nerve root irritation and inflammation. ESIs are also used to treat neck pain that extends into the arms.

Injections of steroid medications into joints can help to reduce pain and inflammation. For example, the facet joints of the spine are a common cause of back pain. Injections into these joints or blocks of the nerves that go to the facet joints can often be very helpful with these pains. This problem is more common in the lumbar spine, but also occurs in the neck.

Trigger Point Injections are muscle blocks. Muscles that are chronically tense or in spasm become tender and painful. The pain triggers more spasm that can develop into a vicious cycle. Injections into the muscle can help to break the cycle.

Nerve Blocks are injections of medication onto or near nerves. The medications that are injected include local anesthetics, steroids, and opioids. Blocks are used to control acute pain (i.e., shot at the dentist or an epidural block for the surgical delivery of a baby). X-ray fluoroscopic guidance is sometimes used to help place the needle accurately.

Blocks can provide periods of dramatic pain relief, which promotes the desensitization of sensory pathways. Steroids can help reduce nerve and joint inflammation and can reduce the abnormal triggering of signals from injured nerves.

Blocks often provide diagnostic information, helping to determine the source of the pain.

Peripheral Nerve Blocks affect the peripheral nerves; nerves beyond the brain and spinal cord. These nerves transmit sensation and motor (movement) control.

Sympathetic Nerve Blocks. Chronic pain conditions often involve malfunctions of the sympathetic nerves. These nerves regulate blood flow, sweating, and glandular function. For example, blocks administered in different areas of the spine help to reduce pain involving the face, arm, hands, legs, and feet.

Physical Therapy (PT) addresses body mechanics (posture), building strength and flexibility through exercise, injury prevention, and utilizes many modalities. These modalities include electrical stimulation, heat and ice therapy, hydrotherapy, ultrasound, and massage.

Biofeedback is used to treat many types of conditions including chronic pain, migraine headache, spinal cord injury, and movement disorders. It is a type of relaxation training and behavior modification. Biofeedback works to control physiological reactions such as muscle tension, body temperature, heart rate, brain wave activity, and other life responses. The therapy requires the patient's intense participation to learn how to control these functions. Biofeedback does not work for all patients.

Electrical sensors, attached to monitoring equipment, are applied to special points on the patient's body. The monitoring equipment feeds back the patient's progress. The biofeedback therapist teaches the patient mental and physical exercises, visualization, and deep breathing to treat their specific disorder (i.e., low back muscle spasms).

Procedures

Intradiscal Electrothermoplasty (IDET) (intra-dis-kal electro-thermo-plasty) is an unproven minor procedure used to treat low back pain. Back pain and sciatica can be caused by degenerative disc disease, which may include disc bulging or herniation. These conditions can cause nerve impingement, inflammation, and pain. During this procedure, under x-ray guidance, a needle is inserted into the affected disc. A special wire is then threaded through the needle into the disc. After the wire is properly positioned, it is heated. The goal of the procedure is to destroy the small nerve fibers that have invaded the degenerating disc. IDET causes the anulus (wall of the disc) to partially melt. This in turn triggers the body to grow new protein fibers to reinforce the anulus.

Radiofrequency Discal Nucleoplasty (new-klee-o-plasty) is similar to IDET. It is an even newer procedure. A needle is inserted into the disc. Instead of a heating wire, a special radiofrequency probe is inserted through the needle into the disc. This probe generates a highly focused plasma field with enough energy to break up the molecular bonds of the gel in the nucleus essentially vaporizing some of the nucleus. The result is that 10-20% of the nucleus is removed which decompresses the disc and reduces the pressure both on the disc and the surrounding nerve roots.

This technique may be more beneficial for sciatic type of pain than the IDET since nucleoplasty can actually reduce the disc bulge, which is pressing on a nerve root. The high-energy plasma field is actually generated at relatively low temperatures so danger to surrounding tissues is minimized.

Pumps and Stimulators
Patient-Controlled Analgesia (PCA) is used to treat post-operative pain. The device is equipped with a pump that is attached to the patient's intravenous line. It is programmed to dispense the correct dose of pain-relieving medication directly into the bloodstream. The patient is given control over pain by operating the PCA with a hand-held push-button mechanism.

Once past the acute pain stage, the patient is switched to oral medication. The doses administered by PCA are smaller and available more frequently. Pain relief is consistent. This helps to prevent sleepiness and weakness allowing the patient to ambulate sooner. It has been proven that PCA reduces the overall amount of medication needed to control pain.

Spinal Pumps are called intrathecal spinal pumps. Intrathecal refers to the fluid containing space that surrounds the spinal cord. The benefit of administering pain relieving medication through a spinal pump is that medications taken orally are diffused throughout the entire body. A spinal pump delivers pain-relieving medication precisely where it is needed. This treatment is only considered when more standard conservative treatments have been ineffective or have caused intolerable side effects.

The pump is surgically implanted under the skin of the patient's abdomen. A catheter is run to the level of the spine where the pain is being transmitted. Medication is pumped directly into the spinal fluid allowing for a much more potent effect on the spinal cord. This drastically cuts down on the amount of medication needed and provides better pain relief with fewer side effects.

The pump is refilled every 1-3 months by inserting a needle through the skin and through a diaphragm on the surface of the pump. Several different medications can be administered this way. Because the system is under the skin, the risk of infection is minimized and the patient can be fully mobile and active.

Spinal Stimulators. Instead of medication to relieve pain, spinal stimulators use electrical pulses on the surface of the spinal cord to reduce pain. The stimulators are similar to pumps in that they are surgically implanted under the skin, but they differ in that electric signals are used to ease pain.

Electrical signals are passed through the tip of the catheter at the precise location near the involved segment of the spinal cord. The result is a tingling over the painful area, which eases the pain. Current theory is that the electrical current input alters the spinal processing of the pain so that the patient's pain is reduced.

The patient is able to control the stimulator by holding a magnetic pulsing device over the skin on top of the implanted generator disk. The stimulator appears to be effective for patients with back and leg pain that did not get better with spinal surgery. There is data that shows that these patients will do better with the placement of a stimulator than they will with repeat surgery.

Conclusion

As we learn about neuroplasticity, we have learned that good pain management starts with prevention -- when possible, physicians should strive to reduce the intensity and duration of acute pain.

When pain does persist, then a multidisciplinary approach is often most effective. In severe cases, when the pain is not responding to usual treatments, then the more invasive techniques, such as nerve blocks, spinal pumps, and spinal stimulators should be considered.

It is not always possible to cure the cause of pain, but it is usually possible to reduce pain and suffering.

Chapter 7

An Integrated Approach to Back and Neck Pain

Gerardo Zloczover, M.D.

Integrated pain management is a new approach to treating acute and chronic back and neck pain. Pain afflicts millions of patients suffering spinal stenosis, degenerative disc disease, osteoporosis, failed back surgery, facet disease, myofascial pain, and degenerative scoliosis. Today patients find that modern medical professionals have a different view of pain. Chronic pain is no longer considered long-lasting acute pain and pain perception is individual to the patient.

Traditional spine care and pain management specialists have merged to form collaborative programs for the comprehensive treatment of pain. Patients find many advantages to these programs including the centralization of medical care with less duplication of services from different medical disciplines. An integrated pain management program educates the patient to understand their pain and to learn how it can be controlled. The patient and specialist work together as partners to determine the best treatment.

Pain Assessment - A pain management assessment begins with the patient's pain history, which includes the location, intensity, and duration of pain as well as factors that alleviate or aggravate the pain. A physical and neurological examination is performed. Further, the patient's medical history and test results are reviewed including radiographs (x-rays, MRIs, etc.).

Multidisciplinary Approach - A multidisciplinary approach means the patient's pain program may include different types of treatment. Treatment is pro-

66

vided by the medical professional that specializes in a specific type of treatment. Medical professionals may include a pain management specialist, physical therapist, rehab specialist, and occupational therapist.

Conservative nonsurgical treatment may include a combination of pain relieving medications, anti-inflammatory drugs, physical therapy, and injections. Alternative therapies include acupuncture, biofeedback, stress reduction, and diet modification. In this chapter different types of injection therapies will be discussed.

Epidural Steroid Injections - Steroid injections are potent anti-inflammatory agents injected directly into the epidural (ep-e-do-ral) space close to the affected nerve roots. The epidural space is the area surrounding the spinal cord and nerve roots. These injections are most effective in the presence of nerve root compression. Scientific studies demonstrate inflammation of the spinal nerves following prolonged compression leads to irritation and swelling.

These injections are most effective when given in the first weeks after the onset of pain. Usually, two to three injections one to two weeks apart are required. Only one injection is given if complete pain relief is achieved. The number of injections is limited to a maximum of three to avoid systemic side effects from the steroids. Side effects are minimal and consist mainly of mild tenderness in the area of injection, which disappears in one to two days.

Sterile Procedure - Epidural steroid injections and nerve blocks are administered in a hospital/outpatient medical facility under sterile conditions. Through an IV, the patient is given medication for relaxation. Numbing medication is injected into the skin area where the injection will be placed. The physician uses fluoroscopy to direct the needle into the epidural space at the appropriate spinal level (cervical, thoracic, lumbar). After the procedure, the patient is moved into the recovery area and monitored for about an hour.

Nerve Blocks are injections of anesthetic, steroid, and/or opioid medication. Nerve blocks are performed to relieve pain and/or to determine if a specific nerve root is the pain source. Anesthetic medications numb the nerves, steroids are potent anti-inflammatory drugs that reduce swelling, and opioids are powerful drugs that fight pain. In some cases, nerve blocks can provide extended periods of pain relief. There are different types of nerve blocks; some are listed below.

Cervical, Thoracic, Lumbosacral Medial Branch Blocks target the medial branch nerves. Medial branch nerves are very small nerves that communicate pain from the spinal facet joints.

Facet Joint Blocks are performed to reduce inflammation and pain and to confirm that a particular facet joint is the pain source. The facet joints are small-paired joints on the back of the spine that provide spinal stability and guide motion in the back.

Selective Nerve Root Blocks are performed to reduce inflammation and pain and to determine if a specific nerve root is the pain source.

Conclusion - During the last decade, pain management has evolved into an integral part of patient care, which has dramatically affected the medical community. Medical professionals have a better understanding of pain. Attitudes are changing, diagnostic protocols have advanced, technology has improved procedures, and there are more medication options. The horizon continues to brighten for patients who suffer pain.

Chapter 8

Spinal Surgery: What You Need to Know

Gregory Gilreath, P.A.-C.

The Myth: ... *the only solution
a spine surgeon can offer is surgery.*

Do you believe that? If so, you will be interested to learn that out of 100 patients seen with back and neck problems fewer than 5% require surgery. This means that 95% can be treated non-surgically.

If your problem falls into the 95% group the course of treatment may include anti-inflammatory medication, an analgesic for pain, physical therapy, or injection therapy. Surgery may be recommended if there is nerve dysfunction, structural instability, tumor or infection, deformity, or if pain is uncontrollable.

In the 5% group ... fewer than 5% requiring back or neck surgery may arouse more concern. Notably incapacitating back pain, inability to move an extremity, leg pain, or loss of bowel or bladder control may be signs of progressive neurological dysfunction. In some cases, surgery may be the immediate treatment.

Keep in mind that surgery is not the perfect answer or cure. Spine surgery has its own risks and is very different from other operations. Not every patient is a candidate for spine surgery. This may relate to the patient's general health.

For example, a patient with a cardiac disorder may be at risk during any surgical procedure. If one back or neck surgery fails, the patient may be advised against additional spine surgery because one failure may lead to another. Smoking or diabetes contributes to failed back surgery. Patients who use tobacco are advised to stop at least one month prior to surgery. Nicotine constricts blood vessels, which slows circulation. Without a healthy flow of blood nourishment is not carried as quickly to healing sites. In addition, bone simply does not grow or mend well when nicotine is consumed. People who smoke or use tobacco are apt to have more spine and general health problems.

At one time spine surgery was reserved for the younger to mid-life populations. Fortunately, attitudes have changed and current research shows that elderly patients do quite nicely. The risks in spinal surgery may be well controlled and the success rate may be as high or higher for older patients.

Sometimes seniors are more motivated to get better than younger patients. Younger patients may have more underlying problems such as those associated with family, employment, stress, and depression. This does not mean that older patients do not share some of these problems, but they often have fewer difficulties.

Modern research reveals the population as a whole is increasing in age. Aging disorders include degenerative disc disease, osteoarthritis (os-t-o-arth-rye-tis), and spinal stenosis (spinal sten-oh-sis). During the next 25 years physicians will be treating an expanding elderly population.

Spine Surgery: The Goal
The goal in spine surgery is to restore the patient to his pre-disease or injury functional level as quickly as possible. This means relieving the patient's symptoms, which usually relate to back, neck, arm, or leg pain. In general, the success rates are very good.

Patient Fear and Apprehension

For many patients the thought of spine surgery (or any type of surgery!) is absolutely frightening. Fear and apprehension are perfectly normal feelings. No one wants to have surgery if it can be avoided. Fortunately, most back and neck surgeries do not need to be performed on an emergency basis. Therefore the patient has time to discuss the procedure, their concerns, and other issues with the surgeon, other physicians, and family.

When Surgery is Recommended

If spine surgery is recommended the spine surgeon will discuss the case and proposed surgical plan with the patient's primary care physician. The primary care physician is often responsible for giving the patient medical clearance to proceed with surgery. Keep in mind – if the patient does not want surgery or wishes to get a second opinion, their decision is always respected.

The Surgical Conference

When a patient's condition warrants surgery the surgeon and often his surgical assistant meet with the patient to discuss the procedure in detail during a special conference. The patient is encouraged to bring a family member.

During the surgical conference the patient's medical history and test findings may be reviewed. The surgeon explains in detail the nature of the patient's disorder, how the surgery will be performed, and expected outcome. Any risks or possible complications that may arise during or following surgery are outlined. The patient is encouraged to ask questions.

During the surgical conference the patient is asked to sign a document called an Informed Consent. An

Informed Consent outlines the surgical procedure and includes the risks and other issues discussed with the surgeon. In most cases the surgical outcome is good with little risk to the patient. However since this is a sensitive area, it is best addressed in written form. From a psychological viewpoint, well-informed patients are less anxious about their surgery.

Some patients want to know if they can go home the same day of the procedure (called outpatient surgery or same day surgery). Outpatient surgeries are procedures that are usually defined as minimally invasive. Some types of procedures will require a stay in the hospital.

Another myth about spine surgery is that a long recuperative period in bed is necessary. This simply is not true. Often the patient is up, out of bed, and walking the day after surgery. Even after complex surgical procedures patients are up, in a chair, and walking the next day. In fact rehabilitation or physical therapy may begin the day following surgery to help restore function and mobility. Many patients are very independent within a short time period after spine surgery, even following elaborate spine surgery.

Pre-Operative Tests tests usually include a chest x-ray, blood work-up, electrocardiogram (electro-car-dee-oh-gram, and urinalysis (yu-ri-nal-is-sis). The nurse reviews the patient's medical history including allergies and medication taken daily.

Hospital/Outpatient Pre-Registration
Prior to the day of surgery, the hospital or outpatient facility will call to schedule an appointment for the patient to pre-register. Pre-registration is a simple process. Depending on where the surgical procedure will be performed (hospital or out-patient facility) a

72

staff member will verify information such as the patient's name, address, social security number, and insurance provider.

Meeting an Anesthesiologist
The patient will meet with a member of the anesthesiology department prior to surgery. The anesthesiologist (an-es-thee-z-al-oh-jist) reviews the patient's medical history and answers the patient's questions.

Modern anesthetics help to keep the patient comfortable and pain free during surgery. In most spine surgical procedures general anesthesia is used. General anesthetics temporarily affect the central nervous system.

Pre-Operative Instructions
The nurse or staff member will provide the patient with a written list of instructions to follow before surgery. These instructions may include how to arrange the home for post-operative care, make plans for transportation home, not to eat or drink anything after midnight, medication instructions, and to leave valuables at home (e.g. jewelry, money).

The Day of Surgery
Upon arriving at the surgical facility, the patient checks in and is escorted to a pre-surgical area to change into a gown. The nurse verifies the patient's name and reviews their medical history including allergies.

Intravenous Line (IV)
The nurse starts an IV allowing medication to be injected directly into the patient's bloodstream. Soon the patient is given a sedative. Some times patients become so relaxed they do not remember being taken to the operating room.

Operating Room (OR)

The OR is a sterile environment with large adjustable overhead lights, a surgical table, and other equipment. During the operation the anesthesiologist monitors the patient's heart rate, blood pressure, and level of sedation. Surgery is a team effort with the surgeon taking the lead. The surgical assistant and nurses support the surgeon and anesthesiologist as needed.

Recovery Room

When the surgical procedure is over, the patient is moved into the Recovery Room. In the recovery room the patient's vital signs are monitored to minimize post-operative complications. During this time the surgeon briefly meets with the family. Although sleepy, the patient may be moved into a regular room if he is to stay hospitalized. A patient who has had same day surgery is released home only after they are fully awake and stable.

Post-Operative Pain is relative. For example, a patient who has endured pain for years may not have the same perception of pain that a patient who has not. Pain may be acute, which means it can be severe but is short-lived. Chronic pain is continuous.

Patient-Controlled Analgesia (PCA)

Following surgery, pain control is administered by oral medications, intramuscular injection, or a newer method called Patient-Controlled Analgesia (PCA). PCA puts pain control in the patient's own hand. PCA is a controlled pumping device that feeds pain-relieving medication through the patient's IV.

The patient simply pushes a button for medication. Since the pump is programmed with a prescribed amount of medication for a specific time period, it is impossible for the patient to become over-medicated.

Walking

Depending on the type of surgery, the patient may be encouraged to walk the day after surgery. Some patients require assistance. Movement enhances circulation and healing. Physical therapy may then be added to help the patient build strength and flexibility. Therapy usually continues on an outpatient basis after release from the hospital.

Going Home

Whether the patient is released the same day of surgery or is hospitalized, he is sent home with written instructions for home care. Necessary prescriptions accompany the instructions. It is always important to follow these instructions. Once home, if any problems develop, call the physician's office immediately.

Conclusion

Spinal surgery has come a long way and continues to evolve and advance. When the appropriate indications are present, surgery can be highly successful.

For more information about types of spine surgery, see Chapter 9, Page 76. If you have Internet access and would like to learn more about spine surgery, and view videos of real surgical procedures, go to:

http://www.spineuniverse.com

Chapter 9

Types of Spine Surgery

Minimally Invasive Spine Surgery

The trend in spine surgery has moved toward minimally invasive procedures. More than 20 years ago a similar trend started with knee surgery. At that time if a patient had torn knee cartilage the surgical procedure required opening the knee. It took several weeks or months for the patient to recover. Now many knee surgeries are performed through small keyhole incisions using an arthroscopic tube. Similar advances continue to be made in spinal procedures. Devices are now available that use microscopic fiber optics that transmit anatomical images to a monitor similar to a television. The equipment is made with built-in magnification that enables the surgeon to view tiny structures through a portal. See Figure 19, Page 162.

Open Surgery versus Minimally Invasive

Spine surgical procedures are often referred to as an open procedure or minimally invasive. Open procedures require larger incisions, muscle stripping, more anesthesia, operating time, hospitalization and, the patient usually needs more time to recuperate. Minimally invasive surgical techniques utilize portals or tiny incisions made in the skin (percutaneous) through which small, specialized instruments are inserted. For example, an endoscope allows the surgeon to see an illuminated and magnified view of the operating field through a tiny incision.

Today many different types of spine surgery can be performed utilizing minimally invasive techniques. Some types of minimally invasive spine surgery use laser technology. Lasers may be used to separate or eliminate tissue. New instruments for use in minimally invasive spine surgery have been developed and continue to be refined.

Discectomy and Microdiscectomy are terms that mean the surgical removal of part or an entire intervertebral disc. The difference between these terms is that microdiscectomy uses microscopic magnification. These procedures are performed to remove a herniated or ruptured disc. The advantage to microdiscectomy is that the procedure is minimally invasive. The incision and instruments are small, which enables the patient to recover quickly.

Interbody Cage Fusion is a newer spinal implant designed to be filled with bone graft and inserted into the empty space created by a discectomy (disc removal). A cage is similar to a tiny birdcage. Bone graft is packed around the cage following implantation. Like instrumentation and fusion, the bone graft grows into and around the cage and creates a stable construct. See Figure 20, Page 163.

Laminotomy and Laminectomy
An easy way to learn the difference between these terms is to remember 'ectomy' means to remove. For example, an appendectomy is the removal of the appendix. Laminotomy and laminectomy are surgical procedures involving the lamina; a thin bony layer covering the spinal canal. The lamina may obstruct the surgeon's view of an intervertebral disc. Laminotomy is the partial removal of the lamina. Laminectomy is the complete removal of the lamina. See Figure 21, Page 164.

If an intervertebral disc has herniated the surgeon may need to remove pieces of the disc compressing nerve roots. With part or all of the lamina removed, the surgeon has a better view of the disc. These procedures also provide greater access to the spinal canal and other parts of the spinal anatomy.

Foraminotomy is a surgical procedure to treat foraminal spinal stenosis. The foramen (small passageways) created between vertebrae provides space for nerve roots to exit the spinal canal. If the foramen is clogged with debris the size of the pathway is reduced and may cause nerve compression, inflammation, and pain. In a foraminotomy the surgeon uses small tools to shave open the inside of the foramen to increase its size. When nerves have ample room, inflammation and pain are relieved. See Figure 16, Page 159.

Spinal Instrumentation and Spinal Fusion

Spinal Instrumentation is a generic term for surgical procedures that use cages, hooks, plates, rods, or screws to stabilize the spine. See Figure 22, Page 165. These devices are made of Titanium alloy and may be called spinal implants or hardware (slang). Instrumentation and fusion may help provide spinal instability and correct deformity. For example, degenerative disc disease may cause instability and progressive scoliosis may lead to deformity.

In conjunction with spinal instrumentation, bone graft is used to facilitate **Spinal Fusion**. Fusion occurs when bone graft grows in and around spinal implants similar to reinforced concrete. Instrumentation and fusion create a strong construct to stabilize the spine. The need to wear a brace following surgery may not be necessary. However, each patient is different and the spine surgeon will decide if a brace is necessary.

The benefits of spinal instrumentation and fusion are numerous. Some implant procedures are performed using minimally invasive techniques. Implants provide

78

the spine immediate stability, which may allow the patient to get up the day after surgery. Before implant use, bone graft simply was not enough to support an unstable spine. The patient would be placed in a plaster cast to hold the spine still until the fusion healed.

Today patients are no longer forced to wear plaster casts following back or neck surgery. When additional spinal support is necessary the physician will prescribe a corset or removable brace (plastic and Velcro™) to restrict movement similar to a splint. Braces are worn on a short-term basis. As soon as an x-ray proves fusion has occurred, the use of the brace may be discontinued.

Instrumentation and fusion will not prohibit the patient from bending, but it will limit a portion of the spine's motion. Standing up and sitting down is seldom affected because most of this motion occurs in the hip joints. The trade-off is acceptable because, following fusion, pain from movement may be reduced or eliminated.

Bone Growth Stimulators are sometimes used in patients who are at high risk for failed fusion (diabetics, smokers). This device is placed internally complete with a battery (similar to a pacemaker) or worn externally like a belt. Stimulators emit electromagnetic waves that 'stimulate' bone tissue to heal. However, just because these devices are available does not mean that all high-risk patients are suited for fusion.

Artificial Discs
The efficacy of artificial discs is now being studied in clinical trials. There are several types being tested including composite discs made of polyethylene, hydraulic discs with a gel-like core that expands, elastic

discs made with a rubber core, and mechanical discs with hinges and springs. The goal of an artificial disc is to replace a faulty intervertebral disc, which is important to the spine as a shock absorber.

Bone Morphogenetic Protein (BMP) is a genetically produced protein with the ability to stimulate a patient's own bone cells to make more bone. This development is especially important to patients who will undergo spinal instrumentation and fusion procedures in the future. BMP has been studied and shown to be safe and effective. Food and Drug Administration (FDA) approval is imminent.

Image-Guide Spine Surgery combines Computer Assisted Surgery (CAS) and the concepts of a Global Positioning System (GPS). This technology enables spine surgeons to view and navigate a patient's anatomy three-dimensionally in real time. This amazing technology allows surgeons to pre-plan spine surgery visually using a computer.

Conclusion

Advancements in spinal instrumentation, fusion, and new technology are constantly improving. To learn more about this subject, see Chapter 12 "Advancements in Spine Surgery" on page 115.

You can also read about other new technologies at *http://www.spineuniverse.com*

Chapter 10

The Cervical Spine:
Degenerative Disorders and Treatment

Steven R. Garfin, M.D.
Christopher M. Bono, MD

Introduction

At one time or another, most people have experienced neck pain. In the vast majority of cases, this is a benign, self-limited complaint. Symptoms are commonly described as a soreness or stiffness of the neck, which may or may not be associated with a minor injury. Patients often attribute this to a "cold wind" or "sleeping wrong" that may or may not be a factor. Most commonly, degenerative disorders of the spine are responsible. Degenerative "disease" is the changes associated with spinal wear and tear or age. Though among the most frequent causes of neck pain, it is the sometimes the most difficult to treat.

Other possible disorders that can cause neck pain are rheumatoid arthritis (room-ah-toyed arth-rye-tis), infection, or cancer. It is rare that such conditions cause only neck pain, as they are usually associated with other warning signs such as profound or unintentional weight loss, fevers, or pain in other joints such as the hip or knee.

The focus of this chapter is a discussion of degenerative disorders of the cervical spine. These affect adult patients of any age, with a tendency for particular disorders to affect certain age groups.

Cervical disc herniations are more characteristic in the young (less than forty-years old), while cervical spondylosis (spon-dee-low-sis) and stenosis (sten-oh-sis) are typically found in older patients. Treatments vary from observation, medications, and therapy to injections or operative intervention.

Definition: Degenerative Disease
As a patient, the first question is obvious. "What is degenerative disease of the spine?" In all honesty, the academic leaders of the spine world are currently pondering this same question. What we mean is that spine doctors can recognize and treat degenerative disorders of the spine but are often unclear how the disorder actually arises except to attribute it to age. To date, most theories about how the spine degenerates remain just that—theories. Although these theories are often well thought out and reasonable, it is exceedingly difficult to prove them. Regardless, it is worthwhile trying to understand them, as they are the best explanation we have to explain degenerative disease of the spine at this time.

Degenerative disease of the spine refers to a break down of the normal architecture of the various components of the cervical spine. Normally, the neck is very flexible. As you may demonstrate on yourself, the neck allows the head to rotate from side to side nearly 180 degrees, to flex forward to touch your chin to your chest, and extend backwards to almost touch the back of the head to your upper back, as well as bend your head toward your shoulder (and all ranges in between these basic motions). These motions are afforded by the various joints of the cervical spine.

There are seven cervical bones in the spine. Known as vertebrae (ver-ta-bray), they can be likened to the cars of a passenger train. The cars of the train, by themselves, are stiff with no ability to bend. Each car (i.e. vertebra) is joined to its neighbor by a joint. The joint allows motion between the cars. As in the spine, joining a number of cars together can allow overall motion. The more joints and vertebrae (the plural of vertebra), the more motion is allowed. In contrast to the joints of the car, the cervical vertebrae are connected by three joints. This gives the spine more stability, while still allowing motion. The extremes of motion must be limited because of the fragile "freight" that the vertebrae hold—the spinal cord. Like the people in the cars of the train, the spinal cord is located in the center of the vertebrae.

At this point, clarification of terms is important. "Spine" refers to the bony parts. These are the vertebrae that were described above. "Spinal cord" is the nerve elements that travel within the spine from the brain down to the rest of the body. The spinal cord transmits signals (bioelectrical and biochemical) that control all the functions (muscles and sensation) below that level. The function of the spine is to protect the spinal cord from injury during motion and activity.

Joints are comprised of two opposing surfaces of bone. Some joints are covered with smooth, glistening cartilage. The slippery properties of cartilage (car-til-ledge) make the two surfaces move easily in relation to each other. The facet joints of the cervical spine have these properties. See Figure 5, Page 148.

In contrast, the main joint between two cervical vertebrae is made up by a large spongy mass, the intervertebral disc. This disc sits between the two broad flat surfaces of the vertebral bodies. See Figure 3, Page 146. The disc is made up of specialized materials that act as a soft "glue" between the bones, while still allowing them to move. The disc is extremely important to spinal stability.However,it is a frequent site of degeneration or breakdown.

In another way the disc can be considered as a pillow in between two bones. The pillows can softly resist the downward forces placed on the vertebrae from the weight and movement of the head. A good pillow is thick and soft and functions best. It allows some movement between the vertebrae. Because the pillow is well fixed to both bones, it resists the tendency of the bones to become misaligned. With time and use the pillow can become flattened.

In this state the disc no longer provides adequate cushioning between the vertebrae. The bones then come closer and closer together. Because the disc is no longer sustaining the forces that it usually does, the other joints of the spine are forced to take on these extra loads. The two smaller sliding joints (facet joints, fah-set) have greater demands placed on them.

Since they were designed to sustain only a small portion of the forces of the spine, the previously glistening, healthy cartilage starts to breakdown. As the cartilage degenerates, the underlying bone becomes exposed and an inflammatory reaction begins. This causes irritation of the joint, which can lead to pain. This sets up a vicious cycle of events. The more the facet joints become degenerated, the less they are able to tolerate the increased demands. Thus, greater demands will then be placed on the intervertebral disc, causing it to further degenerate (or breakdown) as well. The changes in the intervertebral disc and facet joints are not reversible at this time.

Common Disorders
Cervical Stenosis
An important feature of disc degeneration is the reaction that the bone undergoes. Because the normal relationships of the bones are lost, there is a condition of instability. This refers to one vertebra moving in an

abnormal manner in relation to the next vertebra. To attempt to stabilize this excess motion, bone grows outward. These outward growths are called osteophytes (os-t-o-fights). See Figure 15, Page 158. Osteophytes can be found near the disc spaces and around the facet joints. Osteophytes take up space. If they grow in areas where nerves or the spinal cord are nearby, they can impinge or compress these structures. This can cause pain, numbness, tingling, or weakness to varying degrees. If significant enough to cause nerve dysfunction, it is known as cervical stenosis.

Cervical Disc Herniation
Disc degeneration can sometimes follow a slightly different course. In the process of sustaining increased mechanical loads, the outer aspect of the disc, known as the anulus (an-you-lus), can become stressed. With time, small tears can form in the anulus. This outer ring normally keeps the soft, gel-like center of the disc contained. The gel center, known as the nucleus, can be ejected from the disc through an anular tear. This is called a disc herniation (her-knee-aye-shun). If the disc herniates in the direction of the spinal cord or nerve root, it can cause neurologic compromise. Disc herniations in the cervical spine can be serious. If significant enough, they can cause paralysis of both the upper and lower extremities, though this is extremely rare.

In most cases, a patient complains of neck pain associated with radiating pain to one arm. This is caused by compression of a nerve root, rather than the spinal cord itself. With time some herniated discs resolve or shrink by themselves. Sometimes, disc herniations can persist, causing prolonged symptoms and neurologic problems, which may lead to surgical considerations.

Cervical Spondylosis

This rather elaborate sounding word is really nothing more than a description of what happens to the vast majority of our cervical spines as we get older. The term spondylosis (spon-dee-low-sis) refers to the bony overgrowths associated with aging of the spine. Though it is hypothesized, as discussed, that osteophytes form because of micro-instability and disc degeneration, this is not certain. It is known that a high percentage of patients without any neck pain or other symptoms have spondylosis of the spine. In some people, however, spondylosis may be associated with neck pain. Spondylosis is likely the end result of disc degeneration that has been present for a very long time.

Differential Diagnosis
What else can be causing my neck pain?

Diagnosing degenerative disorders of the spine starts with a good history and physical examination. Typically, patients have neck pain. This is the most common complaint. Unfortunately, neck pain is a common complaint in the vast majority of people who have nothing more than a stiff neck. It is important to differentiate neck pain related to degenerative spinal disorders from other more serious ailments.

Muscle strains can cause mild pain. This can vary from the occasional "stiff neck" (from keeping your neck in one position too long like during sleep) to neck soreness associated with a low-speed motor vehicle collision (whiplash). The pain and tenderness is not deep and is usually limited to the surrounding muscles around the neck. Often, one side is more symptomatic than the other. Muscle strains are differentiated from degenerative disorders by their self-limited course. Muscle strains usually resolve, or at least dramatically improve, within a couple of days to weeks. Pain that continues for more than three weeks without improving may not be a muscle strain and other diagnoses should be considered.

Patients with rheumatoid arthritis (room-ah-toyed arth-rye-tis) can have neck pain. It is important to recognize this. Any patient with rheumatoid arthritis should have neck x-rays taken. These patients can develop instability in the upper cervical spine that can endanger the spinal cord. This is easily recognized on plain x-rays.

Neck pain can be a presenting symptom of meningitis, an infection of the brain and spinal cord linings. Meningitis can have many causes and may be contagious. Although neck pain is probably the most common symptom, it is important to recognize the others signs. Patients often are extremely sensitive to light, irritable, have high fevers, and actually tolerate very little movement of the neck. Though it is rare, this diagnosis is very serious and should prompt an individual to seek urgent medical care. Other types of infection can also occur in the neck. Infection can occur in the bone or intervertebral disc. This is more common in older patients who may have a weak immune system. Again, as with meningitis a history of fever could be important, but there is not hypersensitivity to bright light.

Tumors can also cause neck pain. One way to clinically differentiate tumor from degenerative disorders is the presence of generalized, or constitutional, symptoms. Unintentional weight loss, feeling of extreme lethargy, persistent low grade fevers, and night sweats are typical constitutional symptoms. A history of cancer elsewhere is also a clue, as the majority of neck tumors are metastases (or spread) from a cancer in the lung, prostate, kidney or breast.

Typical Cases

Cervical Stenosis

As discussed above, cervical stenosis means, literally, tightening or narrowing of the canal around the spinal cord. Of the degenerative disorders discussed in this chapter, it is potentially the most serious. If the cervical stenosis is profound enough, it can cause dysfunction of the spinal cord known as myelopathy (my-il-lop-ah-thee). The typical person who has cervical stenosis and myelopathy may be in his or her fifties or early sixties. The patient often has complained of neck pain for many years. In some cases, the pain can actually be mild. Therapy may have been prescribed, in addition to medications, for the pain. The other features of this disorder will be demonstrated in an illustrative case.

Presentation. Mrs. S is a sixty-one year old woman with a long-term complaint of neck pain. In the past, her pain has been amply controlled with ibuprofen (Motrin™) and some home exercises. Occasionally, she wears a soft cervical collar to calm her neck spasms. She is an avid knitter and has made several sweaters and scarves for her grandchildren recently. In the past two months, however, she finds that her fingers are becoming clumsy, and she has to take frequent breaks. In addition, Mrs. S is finding that she is not as agile buttoning her shirts in the morning. She is not complaining of any pain in the arms or legs. Interestingly, her legs are a bit wobbly, but she attributes that to some arthritis that has set in over the years. Mrs. S has had no problems urinating on her own, and no change in her bowel habits or control.

Examination. At the doctors' office she is given a full examination. She has a somewhat decreased range of motion of the neck, with some pain at the extremes of the movements. She walks with an abnormal gait, which can be described as "wide-based." In looking at her feet during ambulation, her feet are more spread apart than normal and she stumbles a bit with some steps.

Her reflexes in her arms and legs are very jumpy. This is termed hyperreflexia (hi-per-re-flex-e-ah). She does not have any noticeable weakness in the arms or legs. Because of these findings, the doctor gets some x-rays in the office.

Diagnostic Tests. The plain x-rays show a degenerative spine. As discussed above, this can be better termed as spondylosis. She has osteophytes in the front and back of the spine, which might be protruding into the spinal canal. From the x-ray, there does not appear to be any masses or lesions that would suggest a tumor or infection. Mrs. S's doctor knows that these bony changes are very common at her age. Also, he understands that the plain x-ray is not a very good way of assessing the spinal cord or the space around it.

Mrs. S is sent for an MRI scan of her neck. This test entails her lying down for about forty-five minutes in a long-tube. The long-tube has a very large magnet in it. This is what is responsible for the magnetic part of the magnetic resonance imaging (MRI). Because different tissues in the body respond to magnetic fields in different ways, they have characteristic appearances on MR images.

Mrs. S's MRI showed severe narrowing of her spinal canal. Most of this narrowing is coming from degenerated discs that are protruding into the spinal canal. These discs appear hard and have bony osteophytes above and below them, making the compression even less forgiving.

Specialist Consultation. After getting the MRI report, Mrs. S's doctor sends her to a spine surgeon. She explains to the patient that her condition is called cervical stenosis. Because her stenosis, or tightening, is severe, the nerves in the spinal cord cannot function normally. The compression of the spinal cord is causing her to fumble with her knitting needles and shirt buttons, as well as giving her "wobbly" legs. This surprised Mrs. S the most, as she was sure that she had knee arthritis that was causing her leg symptoms. The spine surgeon explained that the nerves that go to both the arms and legs pass through the neck within the spinal cord. Thus, compression at the neck can cause symptoms in the arms and legs.

Asking what can be done about her condition, the spine surgeon explains that it is likely that her finger and leg fumbling can get worse. In fact, the tightening around the spinal cord can get to a point that she may lose control of her bladder and bowels. In the best case scenario her symptoms will stay the same for the rest of her life, which can be expected in a low percentage of patients.

The treatment options given to Mrs. S are that she can be treated non-operatively or by surgery. The surgeon explains what comprises non-operative treatment. It includes nonsteroidal medications (like Motrin™, Naprosyn™, Celebrex™, or Vioxx™), physical therapy for the neck muscles, cervical collar use, and traction. Of the options, Mrs. S was most concerned about traction, as she would have to be lying down for a portion of the day while the weights were attached to her chin and head.

Mrs. S was also informed of the surgical options. Because of the extent of her disease, the surgeon explained that the best method of relieving the

90

pressure on the spinal cord was to remove the bone from the front of the neck and off the spinal cord. This is known as a corpectomy (core-peck-toe-me).

This would entail an incision in the front the neck through which the surgeon can remove the parts of the vertebral bodies that are compressing her spinal cord. In place of the vertebral bodies, a large piece of bone from her own pelvis, or a cadaver donor, would be inserted. This bone would be expected to heal in place. This is known as a fusion. The likelihood of catching any disease from the cadaver bone is extremely low and is in fact much lower than contracting any disease from a blood transfusion. The more significant risks were from the surgery itself, she was told. The possible complications include damage to the large arteries that supply blood to the brain and to the spinal cord. Spinal cord damage may cause Mrs. S to be completely paralyzed from the neck down. These are the most serious complications; she was informed.

Other possibilities, like infection are also possible, but are more easily treated. Damage to the nerves that supply the vocal cord is also a potential complication. Mrs. S was made aware of this possibility, and that she could have hoarseness permanently after the operation. After hearing the options, Mrs. S asks the spine surgeon a few key questions. First, if she has damage to her spinal cord already, what are the chances of her symptoms getting better with surgery?

Because she is still highly functional, she has a good chance of resolving some, though perhaps not all, of her neurologic symptoms. Her neck pain, though not the focus of the surgery, may or may not get better. If the surgery is a complete success, she will be able to return to her previous activities with a greatly decreased chance of her spinal cord being compressed further. In essence, the surgery is mostly to keep her from progressively getting worse and/or prevent a catastrophic event like a spinal cord injury, which could result with a very minor injury such as a fall or slip.

What will happen to her if she doesn't choose surgery? From the studies available, it is probable that Mrs. S's cervical stenosis will worsen with time. Although it is possible that she could live the rest of her life without any advancement of her problems, it is unlikely. Furthermore, it is even more unlikely for her neurologic symptoms to significantly improve.

"What happens if the piece of bone doesn't heal in place?" This is a rather common complication, occurring in about 15 to 20 percent of patients undergoing this procedure. In the event that the bone doesn't fuse in the front, a second surgery to fuse the back of the vertebra is performed. This is done by an incision along the back of the neck.

Outcome. Weighing the options and contemplating the possible complications of both operative and non-operative treatment, Mrs. S decides to proceed with surgery. Thankfully, the surgery was without complication. After surgery, she remained in the hospital for three days. Her neck was very sore, but strong pain medication helped manage the pain.

She was instructed to keep a hard cervical collar on at all times for six weeks. She was able to get out of bed the day after surgery and started eating a full diet, as she was able to tolerate. After she was discharged, she followed up with her surgeon in the office. The wound healed well. After six weeks she did not use the cervical collar anymore. The bone graft showed good signs of healing to her own bone on the x-rays.

After three months, she felt that her fingers were working better and she no longer felt wobbly in the legs. She returned to knitting, producing a blue baby bonnet for her newborn grandson.

Cervical Herniated Disc
Just as in the lumbar spine, cervical spine discs can herniate and cause pain, numbness, tingling, or even spinal cord compression. Typically, patients complain of neck pain associated with pain radiating to one arm. This is termed radiculopathy (rah-dick-u-lop-ah-thee). Patients who have herniated cervical discs are younger and often more active than those with cervical stenosis. The disc herniation may be associated with a particular incident, such as a sudden jerking movement or positioning of the neck. Both operative and nonoperative methods of treatment can be effective in relieving symptoms.

Presentation. Mr. D is a thirty-five year old man who has a recent onset of neck and right arm pain. He has had neck pain for about six months, while the arm pain is more recent. Mr. D also describes some numbness in the right hand, which he attributes to carpal tunnel syndrome. Though he had never been diagnosed with carpal tunnel syndrome, he seemed to have very similar symptoms as a good friend of his who was recently diagnosed with this disorder.

He is very active, lifts weights and runs about two miles daily before working as an accountant. He does not have any other symptoms. He has no other significant medical problems. Mr. D has no bowel or bladder complaints. He has never sought medical care for his neck pain, which to him is more significant than his arm pain. The arm pain comes and goes, but is tolerable. The neck pain, on occasion, prevents him from going to work. Usually, one day off with a brief course of aspirin works to relieve the pain. Running does not seem to aggravate it and his weight lifting exercises seem to decrease the pain, temporarily. Because of the onset of arm pain, he seeks medical attention, as he feels this might be related to his neck.

Examination. His primary care doctor examines Mr. D. He has near full range of motion of the neck with some mild tenderness along the muscles of the back of the neck. In palpating (feeling) the back of the neck, it seems that he has some tenderness in the midline. The doctor believes this to be in the area of the C5-6 vertebrae. The shoulders, elbows and wrists also have good range of motion and do not appear to have pain associated with their movement.

The neurologic examination demonstrates that Mr. D has some decreased sensitivity of his thumb and along the outer forearm. He does not exhibit any weakness or abnormal reflexes. The remainder of his examination is normal. Because of the numbness and the suggestion of carpal tunnel syndrome by the patient, the doctor orders an EMG, or an electromyography test (elec-tro-my-ah-gra-fee), of his upper extremities.

Diagnostic Tests. The EMG demonstrated what is known as cervical radiculopathy. In brief, the EMG is a test of nerve function in the hands and arms. Based on the distribution of nerve abnormalities, the electromyographer can determine if nerves are being compressed in the hand, elbow, shoulder, or cervical spine. Because nerves are continuous structures, they can also be compressed in more than one location. Mr. D's electromyogram showed no evidence of compression of nerves within the arm itself, but rather that the nerves were being compressed in the spine. This is known as radiculopathy.

With the EMG results, the primary care doctor is now concerned about a correlation between Mr. D's neck pain and arm symptoms. He then orders x-rays of the neck and an MRI of the cervical spine (doctors love to exchange medical words with lay terms—thus neck means the same as cervical spine). Believing that Mr. D may have significant findings on the MRI, he sends his patient to see a spine surgeon.

Specialist Consultation. The spine surgeon examines the patient and agrees with the primary care doctor's assessment. There is definite numbness along the thumb and outer aspect of the right forearm. This is the area to which a particular nerve, C6, supplies sensation. Thus, he would expect to find compression of this nerve on the MRI. Looking over the EMG results, the electromyographer found that C6 nerve root function was altered on the right side compared to the left, an indication that the nerve is being compressed. The plain x-rays did not show any abnormalities and were deemed normal. The MRI, however, was a bit more interesting. The radiologist detected a small herniation of one of the cervical intervertebral discs. The disc herniated on the right side and was compressing the C6 nerve root. There was no compression of the spinal cord, and there did not appear to be any other disc herniations.

The spine surgeon discussed the diagnosis with Mr. D. He stated that what he had was a cervical disc herniation and that this was causing his arm numbness. It has probably been developing over a period of time, and likely explains his six months of neck pain. It is understandable that the disc may have started to degenerate over time and that finally, the nucleus of the disc popped out. This was the time of onset of the arm pain.

Mr. D was a bit confused at this time. Why was the other doctor calling his problem a "radiculopathy" when he really had a herniated disc? In actuality, the surgeon explained, the cervical disc is what is causing his radiculopathy. In other words, the term radiculopathy indicates that the nerve is being pinched. This usually occurs because of a herniated disc, but can happen in other disorders.

Mr. D is now concerned about what to do about his condition. He tells the spine surgeon that he can live with the pain and numbness in the arm, and that he knows what to do for his neck ache when it flares up. Basically, the pain is tolerable. The surgeon reassures Mr. D that if he can tolerate the pain, he can continue his regular activities. If he so desired, he could start a course of physical therapy to strengthen his neck muscles and increase their flexibility, but he is probably doing a good job of it in the gym on his own. The doctor does inform him that good non-steroidal inflammatory medications are available over the counter, though therapeutic doses may vary than written on the package. Additionally, many other medications can be prescribed.

Mr. D was given another non-surgical option called an epidural (ep-e-do-ral) steroid injection. This entails an injection into the space around the spinal cord and nerve roots in the neck. It can be directed to the particular nerve root being compressed by a herniated disc. It is effective in about 60 percent of cases and, as the surgeon explained, is not an unreasonable alternative to surgery.

The surgeon does inform Mr. D of the operation that he could have done. It is called a cervical discectomy (dis-eck-toe-me) and fusion. Similar to Mrs. S's operation, it involves an incision in the front part of the neck to gain access the intervertebral disc. The disc is then removed and a piece of bone graft is placed in between the two bones. This causes the bones to fuse together into one large bone. The same risks and complications are explained to Mr. D, which include paralysis, infection, bleeding, and risk of the bone not healing. Mr. D appeared quite frightened of the procedure and immediately rejected the idea of it. In further contemplation, he asked what benefits the surgery would have. The surgeon also told Mr. D that if the herniation were located more laterally (to the side) another option would be an operation through the back of his neck. This would be a laminotomy (lamb-in-ah-toe-me, removing a small amount of bone) to gain access to the spinal nerve, moving it, and taking out only the herniated component of the disc.

The surgeon explained to Mr. D that the operation, if completely successful, would be most effective in relieving the arm pain and numbness. The relief of his neck pain would be more variable, but he would have a good chance of relieving that as well. The danger of not having the operation is minimal. In other words, what would happen if the disc herniation got worse and compressed the nerves even more? The doctor informed Mr. D that if his weakness got worse, and if he started to have other symptoms like wobbly legs and incoordination of the fingers, that he should return to the office soon. This may be an indication that the disc is protruding farther into the spinal canal and may be compressing the nerves and possibly the spinal cord. If this occurred, the doctor recommends surgery. However, he assured Mr. D this rarely, if ever, occurs.

If the arm and neck pain is tolerable and the nerve function stays the same or improves, there is no need for surgery. This is the option chosen by Mr. D. Since seeing the spine surgeon, he has been taking his medication when he experiences pain. His numbness actually improved over the next couple of months. He has remained active in his jogging and weightlifting, though the latter may not be mechanically as "friendly" to his spine as aerobic exercise.

Cervical Spondylosis

Cervical spondylosis (spon-dee-low-sis) can be thought of as "grey hair" of the spine. This means that if you live long enough (and that may only mean forty- to fifty-years of age in some populations) x-rays of your spine will eventually show signs of cervical spondylosis.

As described above, the term refers to osteophytes (os-t-o-fights), or bony overgrowths, that protrude from the vertebral bodies as well as narrowing occurring across the disc spaces as the disc degenerates. Though they can compress the spinal cord (like Mrs. S) or a spinal nerve root (like Mr. D), the vast majority of these osteophytes do not cause any nerve problems. They are a sign, however, that the disc between the vertebrae and the facets (fah-sets) has become degenerative.

Degenerative discs can cause pain. The mechanism of pain is, unfortunately, not well understood. It is thought to be transmitted by tiny nerve endings that innervate the back part of the disc and facet joints. Degeneration can cause pain from the disc, facet joint, or both concomitantly. Diagnostic efforts are aimed to determine which of these structures are the pain generators. Therapy is directed to relieving stresses being placed on these areas.

Presentation. Mrs. P is a forty-two year old woman who was involved in a motor vehicle accident ten years ago. Since then, her neck has never felt "right." She has frequent neck spasms, which cause her to miss many days of work as an assembly line worker. Mrs. P states her neck pain frequently radiates to the base of her head and down into her shoulder blades. She has no arm or leg pain, no bowel or bladder complaints, and no problems with coordination of her hands or feet.

Mrs. P has taken many pain medications over the past ten years. In the first couple of years, ibuprofen was working adequately. About seven years ago, an emergency room physician gave her a shot of Demerol™, which she felt disagreed with her, but did temporarily relieve her pain. Two weeks later, the pain was back.

Her primary care doctor began to prescribe a mild narcotic, Vicodin™, about three years ago. She takes this on occasion, but she does not like the "spacey" feeling she gets when she takes it. She has had two courses of physical therapy in the past. In describing the therapy she states she was given exercises concentrating on extending her neck. She felt this made her pain worse, despite the therapist's reassurance that this would help relieve the pressure across her intervertebral discs. Mrs. P refuses to go back to physical therapy.

Her primary care doctor has also instructed his patient to use a home traction set up. Attaching to the top of a door, Mrs. P uses upright sitting traction. This consists of a chin-head strap connected to a rope, which runs over a pulley. The other end of the rope has light weights (five to ten pounds) attached, which deliver an upward force along Mrs. P's neck. When she is in the traction setup, she experiences some relief, but it is short-lived. The pain usually returns thirty minutes after she has stopped the traction.

99

Mrs. P also uses a soft cervical collar when she has extreme neck spasms. Again, the relief is temporary. She returns to her primary care doctor for a regular visit and to discuss the options for her excruciating neck pain.

Examination. Mrs. P's primary care doctor performs a careful neurologic exam, which shows no abnormalities of nerve function. Her neck is stiff with a markedly decreased range of motion. She notices that when the doctor was testing extension (head to the back) the pain became much worse.

Diagnostic Tests. Over the years, Mrs. P has had numerous x-rays of the spine. Her latest x-ray showed degenerative changes with multiple osteophytes growing from the front and back of the C5 and C6 vertebral bodies. An MRI of her neck, taken one year ago, showed no nerve or spinal cord compression, but shortening of the intervertebral disc height. This suggests that the disc has become dried and degenerated and that it is not functioning normally. More importantly, there appears to be degeneration of the facet joints as well at the C5 and C6 level. Having treated Mrs. P's painful neck for many years to no avail, her doctor has decided to seek a specialist consultation from a pain management physician.

Specialist Consultation. The pain management doctor reviews Mrs. P's records, chart, x-rays, and MRI. His examination demonstrates that her pain is worse with extension of the neck. He tells her that she has what appears to be degenerative cervical spondylosis at the C5-6 level. Because her neck pain is worse with extension, the doctor believes that Mrs. P has pain associated with facet arthritis.

He suggests that she undergo a series of injections into the facet joints to determine if this decreases her pain. The injections would be Lidocaine™ (a numbing medicine) and corticosteroids (to decrease the inflammation). She agrees with this plan.

The injections into the facet joint of C5-6 gave Mrs. P substantial relief. She has seen the pain doctor two more times over the past ten months since her initial visit. Each time, the facet injection helps her pain dramatically to a point where she can skip taking her pain medicines some days. Unfortunately, the effects have lasted only about three months after each injection.

The pain doctor is confident that her "pain generator" is the facet joints at C5-6 in her cervical spine. He explains to Mrs. P that if the pain continues she might be interested in surgery to fuse these two vertebrae together. This would eliminate motion at the painful joints and hopefully relieve her pain. The doctor explains that the procedure has about a 70 percent success rate in providing long-lasting pain relief. He states that he does not perform the surgery and that she would need to be referred to a spine surgeon.

Mrs. P thinks about her options carefully. Though her pain is continuing, she is not willing to have surgery yet. Because of the temporary relief of the injections, she feels that she has been able to resume, to some degree, her regular activities.

As this is the first time she has had improvement over the past ten years, she would like to postpone surgery for as long as possible. The doctor agreed fully with this decision. Surgery on the neck for neck pain is not nearly as reliable at relieving pain as is surgery on the neck to decrease arm pain.

Conclusion

Degenerative disorders of the spine continue to be a significant cause of neck pain in today's population. Understanding of these problems continues to grow. With that, patients' understanding should follow suit. Affected patients should be aware of the possible treatment modalities, including medication, therapy, braces, selective injections, and surgery.

The best patient is an informed one who understands the natural progression of these disorders, as well as the benefits, risks, and complications of available treatments.

For more information about the cervical spine, disorders, nonsurgical, and surgical treatments, go to: *http://www.spineuniverse.com*

Chapter 11

Minimally Invasive Spine Surgery
Lumbar Discectomy: A Patient's Perspective

Richard G. Fessler, M.D., Ph.D.
Robert E. Isaacs, M.D.
Laurie Rice-Wyllie, R.N., M.S., A.N.P.C.

Introduction

Back pain is an unfortunate problem that will affect essentially all of us at some time during our lives. Most of the time, thankfully, the problem is short-lived. If it worsens to affect the sciatic (sy-attic) nerve, the pain begins to radiate down to the buttock, the hip, and further down the leg. See Figure 9, Page 152. The medical term for this condition is radiculopathy (rah-dick-u-lop-ah-thee), an injury to a spinal nerve. It is commonly known as sciatica (sy-attic-ka) or lumbago; names which bring memories of severe pain to those who have suffered from this ailment in the past. Few things hurt as badly as direct "nerve pain." Once you've felt this pain, you'll never forget it. Like its cousin, back pain, even the majority of radicular pain will end on its own without requiring surgical intervention. For the rare case that will not heal spontaneously, surgery may lay in the future.

This chapter provides an overview of ruptured discs, describing what happens when a disc ruptures, why, and various treatment options for it.

What Causes Back Pain

There are a number of causes of back pain. The spine is a complex structure, with a number of joints and nerves, each of which is capable of producing severe pain.

103

For this reason, generalized back pain is not only common, but also very difficult to treat with directed therapy. When the pain begins to radiate down the leg, a doctor can tell that a certain nerve is affected; then it is possible to direct therapy to a specific target.

The lower back is termed the lumbar (lum-bar) spine. The lowest nerves of the lumbar spine not only make up the sciatic nerve, but also are the cause for the majority of back pain that occurs. The spine not only helps to support the weight of the body, but also allows for trunk mobility. This motion puts strain on the most flexible areas of the back, especially the lowest two disc spaces in the lumbar spine.

The discs are the spongy cushions between the bones of the spine, supplying mobility to the spinal while protecting the bones from repeated stress. It is the constant strain that these discs take that leads to their propensity to rupture. See Figure 4, Page 147.

The disc is made of a hard, fibrous shell, the anulus (an-you-lus), which surrounds a more spongy middle, the nucleus. Repeated stress and injury, combined with weight, posture, and genetics, as well as simple bad luck, can lead to the nucleus rupturing through the anulus. The medical condition that results is a herniated nucleus pulposus (her-knee-ate-ed new-klee-us pul-poe-sis, abbreviated HNP).

The disc spaces are named for the bones that they are sandwiched between. The lumbar spine is made up of five bones, or vertebrae (ver-ta-bray), which ends at the part of the pelvis called the sacrum (say-krum). The disc spaces that most commonly rupture are the lowest two – between the L4 and L5 vertebrae and between the L5 vertebrae and the sacrum. The L4-L5 and the L5-S1 disc spaces are the most commonly

104

injured because, being lowest down in a very mobile area of the spine, the most force is put on them during the course of the day.

When a disc ruptures, a piece of the nucleus pushes through the anulus right where the nerve associated with that disc space lies. Because the nerve is tethered at the point in which it leaves the spine, the disc material compresses the nerve. Compressed nerves hurt. Taking weight off the spine by lying down can alleviate some of the pain. Conversely, sitting or straining, or even coughing or sneezing, puts more pressure on the nerve, thus causing more pain.

For that reason, many physicians recommend bed-rest or light activity during an acute phase of a disc rupture. Pain relievers and/or muscle relaxants are used for symptomatic relief. Clearly, some of the pain is related to inflammation around the nerve. Therefore, patients are often put on steroid packs or anti-inflammatory medications (NSAIDs such as ibuprofen). Steroids tend to help the pain a lot, but because of the side effects, they can only be used for a short period of time. Other nonsurgical treatments include physical therapy and direct injections of steroids near the nerve.

The vast majority of disc ruptures will heal themselves when given enough time. Therefore, much of the treatment is essentially designed to alleviate symptoms while the body heals itself. Given several weeks of these treatments, most patients will be significantly better. It is the exceptional patient who remains in severe pain. When a patient's pain worsens, fails to improve, or when a patient experiences muscle weakness, surgery may then be considered.

Several surgical options exist to treat lumbar disc herniations. Essentially, these options are just variations of the same theme. The classic approach, lumbar laminectomy (lamb-in-eck-toe-me), begins with stripping the muscle off of the back over the area of the disc rupture. A microscopic discectomy (dis-eck-toe-me) begins with the same step, but because a microscope is used, the incision is smaller.

Over the last five years, a novel approach has been developed that does not require cutting the over-lying muscles off of the bone. This approach, Micro Endoscopic Discectomy (MED), has been gaining favor with surgeons and patients alike. When the muscle opening is gently enlarged as opposed to cut, much of the post-operative pain is avoided. With MED, a smaller amount of bone is removed and much of the normal anatomy of the back is left intact. When all is said and done, the latter steps of all these procedures are the same - removing a small window of bone, moving the nerve, and removing the ruptured disc.

MicroEndoscopic Discectomy (MED)
A patient is brought into the operating room and is put under general anesthesia. Some surgeons have chosen to perform MED under local or spinal anesthesia allowing the patient to stay awake through-out the procedure. The patient is turned onto his abdomen and padded into position. A fluoroscope (floor-o-scope, a machine which projects live x-ray pictures onto a screen) is brought in for use during the remainder of the operation. The patient's back is scrubbed with sterile soap, and a sterile field is created. Drapes are placed accordingly, and the surgery begins. See Figures 10-A, B, C, D, Pages 111-114.

The disc space is confirmed using the fluoroscope, and a long acting, local anesthetic is injected through the muscle and around the bone protecting the disc. A half to one-inch incision is made. A thin wire is placed through the incision and lowered until it touches the bone. Progressively larger dilators are brought down on top of one another following the wire. In this manner, the muscle is stretched rather than cut. By the time the 4th or 5th dilator is placed, the muscles are stretched to an opening roughly the size of a nickel. It is through this opening that the procedure is performed. Over the last dilator, a working channel is positioned; this circular retractor holds back the muscles and now the dilators can be removed. The retractor is held in place by a mechanical arm attached to the table.

Finally, the endoscope (en-doe-scope) is attached to the edge of the working channel. The endoscope is a camera about as thick as the ink in a ballpoint pen. It projects an image of the base of the working channel blown up to the size of the TV screen. This allows for microscopic manipulation and removal of the tissues.

When a small amount of muscle is left over the lamina (lamb-in-ah), or exposed bone, this is cleaned off. In order to access the nerve, this roof of bone must be removed; this can be done with a small, high-speed drill or a small bone-biting tool called a Kerrison rongeur. The bone just below the endoscope covers the nerve, as it is about to exit the spine. By removing the bony cover, the nerve can be exposed and then safely moved away. After the bone is removed, the yellow ligament (a rubbery layer of tissue) can be seen which protects the underlying nerves. All the nerves, except the exiting nerve, are grouped together in the thecal sac where they float loosely in spinal fluid.

Care is taken as the yellow ligament is separated and removed, exposing the thecal sac and the exiting nerve root. A very small retractor is placed just on the outside of the root, and the nerve and thecal sac are moved together. Directly below the retractor lies the ruptured disc.

Ruptured disc material has a consistency similar to uncooked shrimp. When a small puncture is made into the tissue covering the disc, the disc will often times begin to ooze out. Various tools are used to remove the ruptured disc and other loose fragments of disc in the surrounding area. No attempt is made to remove the entire disc at that level – that is what is supporting those vertebrae. When completed, the small hole will fill in on its own. The case at this point is essentially finished.

The wound is irrigated with antibiotics. As the scope is withdrawn, your surgeon can see the tissues coming back together. A stitch or two is placed at various levels to hold the tissues together to help healing. Typically, buried stitches are used to close the skin, and none need to be removed at a later date. Commonly, Steri-Strips® (small sterile tape) and a loose bandage are applied to the wound. The patient is then positioned on a stretcher, woken up, and sent to the recovery room. In a few hours, if all goes well, he or she may leave the hospital.

Immediately After Surgery
In order to be cleared to leave the hospital, one must pass a few simple tests. First, a person must be able to handle the post-operative pain on oral medications. Although not severe, there is typically some pain at the incision and some muscle ache, which will linger for a few days.

Even occasionally, as the nerve regenerates, there may be some twinges of pain that run down the leg along the course of the nerve. As long as these twinges do not become frequent events, they are not surprising and will get better on their own. Like incisional pain, the muscular ache will persist for a few days. In fact, it is not infrequent for the back to be sorer a day later. Once again, as long as it is tolerable, it will get better. Apart from pain, the nurses need to be sure that you can take care of your other basic functions at home. This implies that you will be able to urinate (bladder difficulty can occur after general anesthesia), walk, and tolerate food in your stomach.

What To Expect At Home
The first few days you may be more tired than usual because of the anesthesia. Your back will be tender and you may have residual leg pain, tingling, or numbness. Most people will be taking medications for pain and muscle spasm. These medications are taken for approximately two to three weeks and off and on during physical therapy.

Activities and Follow-Up
We encourage you to walk as much as possible. There are many reasons walking is important. First, it will begin your therapy to strengthen your legs. Walking will also help to prevent blood clots, lung congestion, and increase your general feeling of well-being.

You may take a shower four days after surgery. If you have a clear dressing or gauze over your incision, this may be removed three to four days after surgery. Make sure the dressing is removed before you shower. The Steri Strips® stay in place for one to two weeks. Eventually, they begin to peel off on their own.

Lifting is restricted to five to ten pounds for at least two weeks. Using good body mechanics is very important in maintaining a healthy back. You will begin formal physical therapy two weeks after surgery. The course of physical therapy is usually three times per week for six weeks. During your physical therapy, they will increase your weights gradually and begin stretching exercises. You can expect some increased discomfort once you increase your activity. This should go away quickly. If it does not you should let your physical therapist know so modifications in your plan can be made. They will develop with you a home exercise program. Physical therapy is a crucial part of a successful outcome after your herniated disc surgery. Building strong support muscles will help ensure a healthy back for your future.

Most patients will see a health care practitioner at one week for a wound check and six weeks for a final follow up. The final visit is important to assess how you are doing and answer any questions about future activity.

Conclusions
Back pain and radiculopathy are, unfortunately, common problems that will afflict most of us at one time or another throughout our lives. Thankfully, most of these problems will go away within a few weeks. When the pain persists, surgery may be an option. All surgeries directed at a disc rupture require exposing the nerve and removing the extruded disc material. The differences lie in the manner of the exposure and the post-operative pain that the patient experiences. Unfortunately, no surgery is pain-free. All surgeries require a period of recovery, which may be lessened by using less invasive approaches.

Figure 10-A: Operating Room

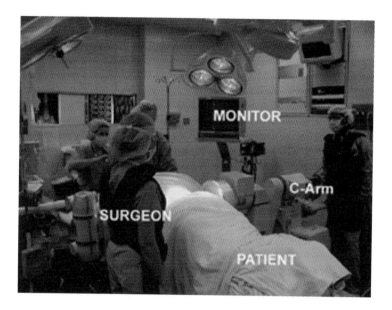

Figure 10-A: Operating Room
An example how the operating room is set-up for a lumbar MED. The surgeon stands on the side of the ruptured disc. The television monitor is across the table. For the majority of the operation, the surgeon performs the surgery while watching it on the screen.

Figure 10-B: Endoscope

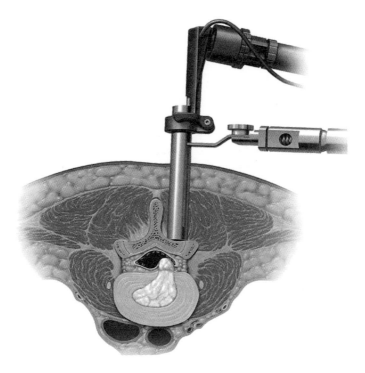

A representation of the working channel once the serial dilators have been removed and the endoscope is placed.

Figure 10-C: Lamina

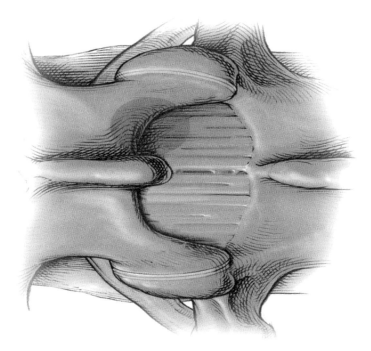

A representation of the area of lamina that needs to be removed to visualize the nerve and the disc rupture.

Figure 10-D: Lamina Removal

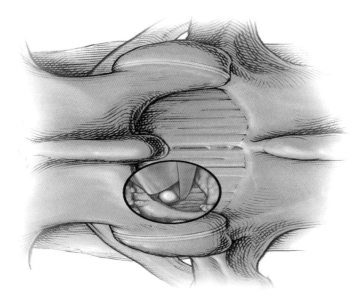

A representation of the intraoperative area and the Kerrison rongeur removing the superior lamina.

Chapter 12

Advancements in Spine Surgery

Gerald E. Rodts, Jr., M.D.

As outlined in Chapter 11 about minimally invasive surgery, the future is bright for new, improved methods of spinal surgery. Other technological and biological advances are on the horizon that will work in concert with minimally invasive techniques.

Several of these, such as computer-assisted image-guided technology, bio-resorbable, flexible and radiolucent spinal implants, and genetic-engineering of disc tissue, bone fusion, vertebral bone, and other steps forward, are worthy of discussion.

Spinal Navigation Technology
Conventional surgery of the spine often involves taking an x-ray during the procedure to confirm the location of the spine or to confirm satisfactory placement of spinal implants (e.g. screws, rods, hooks, plates). Often, surgeons use "live" x-rays during surgery (called fluoroscopy, floor-ah-sko-pee) to obtain this information.

In the past decade, great advances have been made that has taken navigation of the spine (or localization) to a new height. Also known as "computer-assisted, image-guidance," navigation technology is advancing at a rapid rate. More powerful and elegant than simple x-ray technology, spinal navigation technology uses a computer and radiographic studies (x-rays) of the patient to allow the surgeon to know precisely where he/she is at all times.

115

Spinal navigation technology enables the surgeon to more accurately place spinal instrumentation, perform decompression (e.g. eliminate pressure on nerves), remove tumors, and other tasks.

Three-dimensional models of a patient's own spine appear on a computer screen with virtual representations of real surgical instruments that the surgeons have in their hand. Surgeries can even be planned 'virtually' on the computer before a patient even goes to sleep under anesthesia. For example, screw diameter, length, and other measurements can be made with greater accuracy.

The future of spinal navigation is exciting. Rather than send a patient for an preoperative CT or MRI scan, in the future surgeons will be able to obtain images in the operating room that can instantly create computer models of the patient's spine. These models can be used to help navigate the spine during surgery. Intraoperative CT, MRI, and fluoroscopy-based CT offer great potential. The end result is enabling the surgeon to visually "travel" in and out of a patient's spine on computer, thereby allowing them to see things that the human eye cannot during a typical surgery. As spinal navigation technology advances, newer minimally invasive techniques will become available.

Future Biomaterials for Spinal Implants
Titanium
Great success has been achieved thus far using cages, rods, screws, hooks, wires, plates, bolts, and other types of spinal implants made from stainless steel and (more recently) titanium metal. The great advantage of titanium is that it allows for better CT and MRI imaging to be performed after implantation with little interference. Stainless steel causes significant "blurring" of CT and MRI images.

Bone Graft

Other types of materials used in spinal surgery include bone graft. Bone is either harvested from the patient's own body (autologous bone) or bone from a bone bank can be used. Bone bank bone (allograft) comes from cadavers and is commercially processed for transplantation into patients. One problem is bone taken from the patient's pelvic bone (ileum) can cause chronic pain; the other is the supply of cadaver bone can be limited.

Bone Morphogenetic Proteins (BMP)

Molecular biological advances will tie in with these navigational and biomaterial advances. Very soon, genetically-engineered proteins called Bone Morphogenetic Proteins (BMP) will be commercially available for bone fusion surgery. This will likely eliminate the need for either autologous or allograft bone use and all of the potential morbidity and limitations inherent in these grafts. BMP can be placed inside a collagen (protein) sponge or other ceramic-type implants and used instead of bone in areas of desired fusion (e.g. disc space, backside of the spine). Thus, in the future, we may be using biodegradable spacers or "fusion carriers" that house BMP, allow for a solid fusion, and then dissolve away themselves leaving only fusion bone behind.

Ceramic and Carbon Fiber

Other materials have been used as carriers of bone graft or vertebral body replacements such as ceramic and carbon fiber.

Carbon fiber is radiolucent, which means that implants made of this material do not show up on x-ray. This has the advantage of allowing the bone fusion to be better seen. Future developments will bring even greater advances.

Plastics and Polymers

Because of the potential morbidity of using a patient's own bone (autologous bone) and the limited supply of cadaveric bone, attention has been directed to developing newer materials to serve as spacers and conduits for bone graft material. Other forms of plastic are being developed such as polyether ketone combinations that will be radiolucent yet provide strength and support.

Polylactic Acid (PLA) polymers are also being developed that can actually biodegrade over time. In other words, the PLA will do its job in holding bone graft material and providing support long enough for a fusion to take place, and then it slowly dissolves (hydrolyzes) away after a year or so. Still other materials are being developed that would allow some flexibility and dynamism in a spinal implant. There is some agreement that certain spinal implants may be too rigid and more natural, flexible substances may be a better substrate from which implants could be made.

Disc Replacement or Disc Regeneration

In the future, disc replacement or regeneration may replace the role of fusion in some patients. Though fusion will likely always be a very useful form of treatment in many patients, there may be some patients that will benefit from an implantable artificial mechanical disc. Several forms of artificial disc implants have been used in Europe and are currently being tested in clinical trials in the United States.

The theoretical advantage is that artificial disc replacement will result in improved pain and function with maintenance of some motion at a disc space that otherwise may have been fused solidly by more conventional techniques. Other forms of disc replacement may involve re-establishing the inner nucleus of the disc only with a gel-like material and utilizing the natural anular lining of the disc to contain it (without a metallic component).

Equally as exciting is the possibility that genetically-engineered cells may be surgically implanted or injected into a degenerated disc, allowing for regeneration of disc material that can serve as a shock absorber like the disc we are all born with. There is some experience already with the use of engineered cells in reproducing knee cartilage, so the possibility of use in the spine is real.

Summary
Great advances in just the past decade have allowed physicians to treat spinal disorders more effectively. Further advances in biomaterial development, computer-assisted image-guided technology, molecular biology of bone and disc will all be integrated together to develop very powerful techniques for treating spinal disorders. It is this integration of emerging technology and biological advances that will result in smaller incisions, less trauma to normal tissues, faster healing time, equivalent or better relief from pain and neurological problems, and quicker return to functional status.

Chapter 13

What Can Physical Therapy Do for Me?

Dana L. Davis, M.P.T., M.T.T.

A few questions that are commonly asked a therapist include the following -- •What is Physical Therapy? •What can a Physical Therapy program do for me that I cannot do on my own? •How long is it going to take? •Who benefits from Physical Therapy? •What will I have to do in my therapy? Each question is answered and expanded upon below.

What is Physical Therapy?
Physical Therapy (PT) is considered a conservative treatment method addressing the treatment, healing, and prevention of injuries and disabilities. Physical therapists focus primarily, but not solely, on relieving pain, promoting healing, restoring function and movement, and facilitation and adaptation associated with injury.

Therapy also focuses on ergonomics or body mechanic training, fitness and wellness and, especially education. This area of physical therapy includes posture, stabilization and building strength in the weakened area, and to prevent additional injury.

What can a PT program do for me that I cannot do on my own?
Many patients may think that they know how to properly exercise, manage their pain and rehabilitate themselves. Patients commonly give therapists reasons why they do not need therapy – for example, "I have had this before and I know what works for me" or, "I know what is causing this because my

neighbor had the same thing, so I will just do what she did" and attempt to self-manage their condition.

A Physical Therapist is a specialist specifically educated and skilled in proper rehabilitation. Physical therapists are continually educated as to management for different dysfunctions, differentiation of one dysfunction/injury from another and work closely with the referring physician in the development of a rehabilitation program specifically designed for each individual patient. The other important aspect to remember with physical therapy is that each individual is different. We all have different types of bodies, different patterns of movement, different alignments and different habits. A physical therapist, along with trained staff, monitor each individual and attempt to correct improper habits, alignments and movement patterns.

Most important with therapy is education. Due to healthcare guidelines and reimbursement changes, your physician may not have the time needed to explain exactly what your injury/dysfunction/disability is and why/how it occurred. Your therapist specializes in this and many times will be the one to educate you on the specifics of your problem and what the course of action will be to correct it and hopefully prevent it from reoccurring. PT focuses on education, correction, and prevention.

How long is it going to take?
This is a popular question. Everyone has other priorities in their day and life. Exercise and therapy can sometimes seem an imposition. The patient has to remember that recovery from injury can be much more time consuming than prevention. Each person's degree of injury is different and will experience a different rate of recovery. In most cases, your

therapist will have an idea as to your personal rate of healing within two weeks. Other factors that play into healing progression and rate of recovery are patient compliance and dedication. Therapists are healers and teachers. However, if the lessons, which we teach, are not practiced and learned, the rate of healing or re-injury is affected.

Who benefits from PT?
Many and all can benefit from therapy. As an active therapist, I work out and am always observing others. I very rarely come across individuals with perfect body mechanics, training techniques, or movement patterns. This is where wellness comes into play. Typically the most appropriate patients are those who have been in accidents (work-related, automobile, or falls), athletes with overstress injuries, arthritic patients, pre and post-operative patients, and those with general de-conditioning, or strains.

Posture is an area that always seems to be overlooked. Patients who make simple changes throughout their daily habits can change their potential for injuries and alleviate current ones. See Figure 18, Page 161.

Standing. When standing, think about what is comfortable. Think about what your mother used to say, "Stand up straight and don't slouch!" Good standing posture involves upright positioning; shoulders back, chin neutral, abdominal muscles tight, arms in line with your body and one foot slightly in front of the other, with knees slightly bent. This is called active posture. It requires muscles to work with the skeletal system for energy conservation and bone and joint protection.

Sitting. When sitting, eyes should be level and in a position such that the neck is neither bent forward or backward. Shoulders should be level and relaxed (without being slumped forward) with appropriate support throughout the spine. A chair should maintain all natural curvatures. Hips and knees should be level with each other and ankles should be vertical to the knees.

Lying. Proper lying positions are those in which the joints are in neutral positions (neither bent excessively forward or backward). The muscles should be supported yet relaxed. Elbows, wrists, hips, and knees should be slightly bent. Too many pillows can be bad. Often too many pillows cause the neck to "hyperflex," which applies too much pressure to the brain's blood supply.

Results of **Poor Posture** may include the following: forward head, rounded shoulders, excessive lordosis (lor-doe-sis, envision a Dowager's Hump or posture associated with chronic cane dependants), tight and weak back muscles, tight and weak leg muscles, which can all lead to joint pain.

What will I have to do in PT?

Therapy generally encompasses pain relief, strength and flexibility training, proper postural alignment, regaining movement or range of motion, improving and correcting posture, endurance training, relaxation and stress relieving techniques, balance and coordination training, proper walking, education, safety awareness, and development, and implementation of a home exercise program.

PT is Worth Your Effort

Remember that each individual is different. Your rehabilitation or PT experience will be individual. Be patient with yourself, your physician and your physical therapy staff. Healing takes time, diligence and compliance. If you think you may be a candidate for physical therapy, speak to your physician or therapist.

Physical Therapy Treatments
Aquatic Therapy
Many patients with osteoarthritis (os-t-o-arth-rye-tis) have found exercising in water to be beneficial. A pool offers a gravity-free environment allowing the patient to perform simple exercises without stressing painful joints. Movement increases circulation to affected joints and can help to relieve stiffness. For some patients, swimming is a good exercise to loosen up stiff joints and strengthen muscles.

Electrical Stimulation ('Stim') forces a muscle or muscle group to contract and relax. The therapist places a pair of surface patches containing electrodes on the skin over the area to be treated (e.g. low back). Each patch attaches to a lead (insulated wires) connecting to equipment that controls and regulates the stim. The therapist programs the equipment to deliver the correct amount of stimulation for a set period of time. The electrical current affects nerve and muscle cells, which may be at rest or reacting to the stimulus.

The treatment is not painful. The patient feels a gentle pulsating or on and off sensation. During this treatment circulation is stimulated supplying the target area with oxygen and nourishment necessary for healing. Physical Therapists have used electrical stimulation for more than 15 years to enhance healing, alleviate swelling, and pain.

Heat and Ice
Heat increases circulation, decreases stiffness, pain and muscle spasm. Patients with early signs of arthritis often find substantial relief from symptoms by taking a warm bath or hot shower. This is best done early in the day to help loosen up and alleviate stiffness commonly associated with forms of arthritis (e.g. osteoarthritis).

Physical therapists use moist hot packs wrapped in several layers of toweling that is laid or wrapped around the effected area. Unlike a heating pad that only delivers surface heat, a moist hot pack transfers moist heat that penetrates deeply into soft tissues and stimulates local circulation more than heat alone.

Ice decreases pain by slowing the speed of nerve impulses. Inflammation, the body's vascular response to injury may subside with forms of cold therapy. Cold reduces the temperature of tissue beneath the skin. Cold packs, ice massage and iced towels are usually recognized as the first aid following trauma. Application of cold therapy for an extended period of time can harm the skin. Treating with ice should be supervised by a physical therapist, especially when treating an overworked body part.

Hydrotherapy is probably one of the oldest therapeutic treatments. Hydrotherapy is similar to a whirlpool bath. Whirlpool tanks are available in different sizes. Some are designed to accommodate the entire body. During hydrotherapy both the water temperature and agitation are controlled for maximum benefit.

Myofascial Release (my-o-fash-e-al release) improves circulation, decreases muscular tension and increases range of motion. Myofascial release is a form of localized massage affecting the muscle fascia. Muscle and groups of muscle are encased in sheets of fascia. During myofascial release, the fascia is manipulated by hand to systematically stretch the tissue. Scar tissue or tight tissue may be loosened using cross friction motion during massage therapy.

Ultrasound is a common treatment and has been in use for more than 40 years. It produces high-frequency sound waves that pass through the skin to promote deep warming of soft tissues (e.g. muscle). The warming effect enhances circulation and healing. Ultrasound is often used to treat muscle spasm and to relax tight muscles. Unlike a hot pack, ultrasound works without harming the skin. The equipment controls the speed and duration of the sound waves.

Movement and Conditioning

All exercise is supervised by a physical therapist responsible for teaching the patient how to move properly while pushing beyond pain thresholds. Physical therapists want patients to work within a pain free range. This does not necessarily mean exercise will be easy in the beginning. Remember the adage anything worthwhile is worth working for.

Warming-Up the body may be accomplished by riding a stationary bike followed by light stretching. Of course the type of warm-up and therapy is dictated by the patient's individual treatment program. Temporary muscle soreness 24 to 48 hours following exercise therapy is normal and should be expected. As regular exercise continues discomfort will subside.

Stretching helps to increase flexibility. Resistive and strengthening exercises may be added as the patient progresses. Some patients are not able to move the affected area without assistance. The physical therapist will then manually move the affected area (e.g. arm, leg) to increase range of motion.

Home Exercise

Physical therapy often includes a customized home exercise program. The instructions may include written and illustrated exercises. Always consult the therapist before starting or changing a physical therapy exercise program. If necessary, changes can be discussed with the patient's physician.

Posture and Body Mechanics

Learning to use proper body mechanics is important to prevent further injury. If the patient is willing to maintain an adequate level of physical fitness, reduce stress, and use proper body mechanics, the risk of injury from activity can be reduced.

Proper posture means maintaining the natural curve of the spine or neutral spine. Good posture helps to minimize stress to the spine. Posture may be the first lesson a physical therapist teaches the patient. Poor posture and body mechanics are two of the leading causes of neck and back pain.

Good posture means the shoulders are held slightly back and level, the ears are in line with the shoulders, the chin is slightly tucked inward, and the pelvis is shifted forward allowing the hips to align with the ankles. Figure 18, Page 161 demonstrates proper posture. Notice the plumb line hangs directly from the ear lobe down the middle of the arm to the ankle.

Avoid Stressful Work Habits

Avoid leaning over the desk for long periods of time. Don't sit too far from the work area without the back supported. *Adjust* the chair height so the knees are bent at a 90-degree angle. *Bend* the elbows at a 90-degree angle; elbows may rest on the work surface. *Avoid* cradling the telephone against the ear and shoulder.

Lifting and Carrying Tips

First, take a look at the object to be moved. If it appears to be too heavy or cumbersome, find help. *Remove* obstacles in the pathway before lifting the object. *Think* about how you will maintain good posture. Get as close to the object as possible. *Place* the feet slightly apart and flat on the floor. *Bend* at the knees to provide a stable base of support. *Tighten* the stomach muscles, keep breathing and smoothly lift the object using the arms and legs – not the back. Try to *hold* the object at the side and bottom. Keep it close to the body with the back straight and carry the object with the elbows slightly bent.

When carrying shopping bags or luggage, split the load in two. Try to carry the same amount of weight in each hand.

Push or Pull?
Pushing is usually more efficient. Keep the back straight and use the knees to push. Stay close to the object by repositioning the body from time to time.

Reaching Tips
Consider the size, weight and location of the object. Use a stable stool or ladder to get as close to the object as possible. Stand on the stool or ladder with both feet flat. Try to directly face the object. One hand could be used for additional support. Avoid looking overhead as this could cause neck strain. Consider storing often-used items within easy reach.

Conclusion
The therapies discussed in this chapter represent those that are often referred to as conservative. In the following chapter, Traditional Chinese Medicine and Back Pain, learn about popular alternatives to physical therapy.

Portions of this article have been reprinted with permission from *spineuniverse.com*

Chapter 14

Traditional Chinese Medicine (TCM) and Back Pain

Laurie Morse, L.Ac., Q.M.E.

Why do so many suffer from pain, specifically low back pain? This is a question that patients and doctors ask with varying degrees of frustration. I'd like to provide an alternative angle of understanding low back pain through the model of Chinese medicine.

Traditional Chinese Medicine (TCM) is a system of medicine that has been practiced for several thousand years in the Orient and has gathered more acclaim in the last decade here in the West.

TCM encompasses the modalities of acupuncture (ak-u-punk-chur), herbal medicine, moxabustion (mox-ah-bust-shun), Tui Na (twee-nah) or medical massage and often includes nutritional therapy and breathing therapy, or Qi Gong (chee-goong).

In November of 1997 the National Institute of Health published a consensus statement stating there is, in fact, sufficient evidence to support the use of acupuncture (for some conditions).

Though, further study of its physiology and clinical value was encouraged, promising results emerged regarding the efficacy of acupuncture in low back pain. I'd like to also note that the use of acupuncture does not preclude the concurrent use of Western medical therapies and often, both are utilized to successfully treat a patient.

The Theory of Traditional Chinese Medicine

When an individual is diagnosed with a "back problem" in Western medicine be it spondylosis (spon-dee-low-sis), spinal osteoarthritis (os-t-o-arth-rye-tis), prolapsed lumbar disc, or muscular/ligamentous lumbar strain, the focus is primarily on the lower back region and within the Western medical model the options become therapies like spinal surgery, physical therapy, pharmaceutical intervention, and cortisone or epidural (ep-e-do-ral) type injections. These are perfectly acceptable modalities but what if they don't alleviate the pain? And, what about the underlying cause for the back weakness in the first place? Can that underlying weakness be strengthened? Let us consider this possibility via Chinese medicine.

Though the system of TCM is logical and scientific in it's own way, it is a separate system from modern Western medicine and can't always be explained via Western medical logic. To include the successful system of TCM within our minds, we need to expand the way we think and consider both systems as valid while learning how to accept the similarities and differences within the two systems.

One could say that Chinese medicine was born out of the theory of Yin and Yang. As well as describing that which exists in nature, Yin and Yang perfectly describes all the parts and functions of the body. Yin and Yang are in a constant state of dynamic balance, when this balance is threatened disease is possible.

An example in nature of this dynamic balance is the rhythm of the sun (Yang) and moon (Yin). In a 24-hour period each is unique, change over to the other and require each other for overall balance (from the perspective of earth that is).

Yin and Yang each have an individual expression in the body and yet requires the other to exist, for example Yin represents stillness, form and blood whereas, Yang represents activity, function and Qi (chee). Qi needs blood to nourish it and blood needs Qi to move it.

Qi can be described as energy, material force, electromagnetic current, matter, ether, vital force, or life force. Qi travels throughout our entire body in channels or meridians reaching every aspect of our body. These channels are understood to be separate from the pathways of the nervous, vascular, and lymph systems in Western medicine.

Loosely, when we are born we begin with a gas tank of Qi and when the tank of Qi is empty our life force is gone or in other words, we die. This tank of gas is rooted in the organ system of the Kidneys according to Chinese medicine theory and is distributed throughout our organs, glands, and channels in a very systematic way.

Because of this intricate channel system within our body when we refer to an organ such as the Kidneys, that includes much more than the organ alone according to anatomy.

Each organ system has representations of Yin and Yang, hormone balance, as well as specific Qi and blood functions, which play a vital role in connecting, via the channels, with other organ systems and the entire body to render the body a holistic system.

In other words, it isn't possible, within TCM, to deem an organ or body part as an isolated problem without considering the whole body system. So, you say, what might this have to do with low back pain?

The Relation of the Kidney System in TCM and Low Back Pain

The low back is the "mansion of the Kidneys" meaning that the low back is most closely related, but not limited to, the health of the Kidney system. It is without question, in low back pain, that the Kidney system be treated in Chinese medicine.

Back on the subject of Qi, it is said in Chinese Medicine:

If there is free flow, there is no pain;
If there is no free flow, there is pain.

Basically, what this means is if the Qi and/or blood stagnate in the channel(s), specifically through the region of the low back, there will be pain. Imagine a river flowing unimpeded and suddenly a tree falls across the river, we see in our imagination the water no longer flowing freely, but getting blocked by the log, pushing into the banks of the river. The basic concept of acupuncture is to re-open the river, create a circulation so that the log lifts and normal flow is restored.

How does the free flow of Qi and blood in the body become impeded, so as to cause pain? An external invasion of wind, cold, dampness, or heat may invade the lower back region causing pain. If our defensive Qi or immune system is weak we become more susceptible to external invasions through the pores of our skin. The Qi and blood can stagnate due to trauma (i.e. lifting, repetitive strain over time, an accident, or similar sprain).

There may be an insufficiency of Qi or blood creating a sluggishness or stagnation of flow throughout the channel(s). This is an internal cause or weakness with a number of possible etiologies such as:

Poor diet, insufficient rest coupled with too much activity or overwork (i.e. busy lives, excessive sex*), overuse of drugs, chronic illness, heredity weakness, an excess of the emotions fear and anxiety, and general aging as our Qi is naturally declining.

*The Chinese believe that a healthy, moderate amount of sex supports a good flow of Qi and too much sex (specifically ejaculation for men and childbirth for women), depletes the Qi, blood and essence of the Kidneys.

Care for Your Low Back According to TCM
Acupuncture
The use of thin, pre-sterilized, disposable needles to re-establish the proper flow of Qi and blood through the channel(s) of the back. This flow increases circulation allowing for oxygen, blood and lymph to support the body's healing process. If the channels have been blocked for a long period of time, or if there is pronounced deficiency of Qi and blood, it is necessary to have acupuncture for a longer period of time to assist the body in regaining it's normal function.

Research has shown acupuncture to cause the release of neuro-chemicals such as: endorphins, enkephalins, serotonin, and corticosteroids all of which contribute to the reduction of pain and inflammation.

Moxabustion
Concentrated herbs that are sprayed or burned above the skin to open and warm the channels.

Herbal Medicine
The use of herbs from the Chinese herbal pharmacopia also dates back several thousand years. Typically, individual herbs are put together synergistically to create a formula with a specific function (i.e. open the

channels or strengthen the Kidneys). Herbs go to specific channels and have specific properties (i.e. sweet, bitter, cold, warm etc.).

Tui Na or Chinese Massage

Working on the meridians with the hands, using techniques specific to Tui Na. Care must be taken not to exacerbate inflammation if it is present.

Proper Diet

If we put vinegar in our finely tuned automobile it won't run. It needs good clean gas. Our bodies' "gas tank" needs good clean nutrients. This means a balance of quality protein, good/essential fats, and carbohydrates (five to nine servings of vegetables and fruit with a moderate of whole grains).

This means no overeating as our body has a hard time managing the overload, eat meals at regular times, do not eat late at night, minimize or eliminate sugar, processed foods/drinks, alcohol, and don't eat any one thing in excess (i.e. dairy products or bread). Drink plenty of water. Contemplate the fact that our body can only be as healthy as the fuel we give it.

Qi Gong Breathing

Qi Gong is the art of therapeutic breathing. Breath is Qi, Qi is life. The two substances that fill our Qi tank up are air and nutrients (breathing and healthy foods). To take in a full breath of air into our abdomen is health promoting, yet poor breathing habits have left most of us breathing on the shallow side.

To begin with make an effort to remember to breathe deeper, post little notes if necessary that say, "breathe deep." Be aware of inhaling fresh air/Qi in through your nostrils all the way down into your abdomen and exhaling through your mouth. Your abdomen should visibly push outward on the exhale and contract back in on the inhale. As well, there are specific breathing exercises to open the spine, which in turn, supports the flow of cerebral spinal fluid. You may want to get a book or video on breathing exercises to support your health.

Deep breathing has far reaching affects in our body by balancing our nervous system, increasing oxygen delivery and keeping the Qi moving. Do not underestimate the value of this simple, yet powerful practice; we have to breathe anyway, why not do it right?

Proper Exercise
Exercise promotes the normal flow of Qi and blood. Our bodies were designed to move. I don't believe it's a coincidence that back pain is on the rise in proportion to an increasingly sedentary lifestyle. Regular aerobic activity, regular stretching, keeping the abdominal muscles strong, and proper body mechanics when bending and lifting are some of the necessities in back maintenance.

Stress Management
Well, this could be an article in and of itself. It has been proven that prolonged stress creates disharmony on many levels: physically, emotionally and spiritually. Explore avenues to keep stress at a minimum.

There is an interesting book written by Robert Sapolsky (a professor of science at Stanford) entitled, "Why Zebras Don't Get Ulcers." He depicts with detail and humor, the effects of stress on our body. I recommend it to anyone interested in understanding and successfully managing stress. Learning to meditate is another recommended way of managing stress as well as pain.

Proper Rest

Our physiology needs regular sleep and rest balanced with the activity we perform. Rest is Yin, activity is Yang, and attention to both is required to maintain balance. When we push ourselves too hard for too long and ignore the need for rest our Yang consumes our Yin and imbalance ensues. A healthy body can recover from a temporary period of hard work or emotional strain; the imbalance only begins when it goes beyond temporary.

What to Expect in an Acupuncture Treatment

Acupuncture is strictly regulated via individual state medical licensing boards as well as the National Committee. Practitioners are typically qualified and trained to provide you with a successful experience. Acupuncture doesn't "hurt" but you may feel sensations that are "different" (like tingling, dull, achy). These sensations are Qi.

The thin needles are inserted according to your individual diagnosis and are left in for approximately 20-40 minutes. During this time, most people experience a deep sense of relaxation, in part because of the endorphins that are released during acupuncture.

Depending on whether your pain is acute or chronic guides the number of treatments you may need. Your pain may be resolved in a few treatments or it may take several courses, in some cases acupuncture serves primarily as pain management. In any case, your whole body benefits from the affects of acupuncture.

I encourage you, if you haven't already, to consider including Chinese medicine as you journey toward a more pain-free and healthier life.

SpineUniverse.com, Used with Permission

Chapter 15

Spine Patients and Internet Use

Gerald E. Rodts, Jr., M.D.

Use of the Internet has grown at a remarkable rate over the past few years for business transactions, entertainment, research, and general communication. One of the most common reasons people access and search the Internet is for medical information.

There are many aspects of the Internet and electronic communication with which all patients must be familiar. When properly used, the Internet can provide significant education for patients and, perhaps more in the future, will provide improved communication between patient and physician, physician-to-physician interaction, and other professional resources for physicians. Searching for medical information on the Internet, however, can be like searching for a needle in a haystack.

Perhaps the most important thing patients need to know when surfing the Internet for information is that there is no governing force or entity ensuring the quality or validity of any site. If one types in the words "spine" or "back pain" or "neck pain" into any search engine (e.g. AOL, Yahoo, MSN, Askewest, About.com), a wide variety of sites will be listed. Some may be advertisements for a particular product, group practice, hospital, pharmaceutical company, physical therapy center, or personal website of an individual.

The Internet surfer must develop a critical eye when viewing any site purporting to offer medical information. The following tips may be helpful.

137

Locating Legitimate Information

If you are searching for legitimate, valid information, take a look at the site's banner and check for a mission statement. A mission statement should briefly describe the goal of the site. If a single corporation or practice sponsors the site, it should be readily apparent. One should realize the potential for bias in any material presented.

Also, look to see if physicians are involved in providing the content of the site. Most sites that boast a "faculty" or "editorial board" of physicians will provide their names and backgrounds that can be checked. In the field of spine surgery, one would want to see names of board-certified neurosurgeons, orthopedic surgeons, physiatrists (rehabilitation medicine), physical therapists, anesthesiologists, registered nurses and nurse practitioners, psychologists and psychiatrists, and neurologists.

Look over the mission statement or informational pages to see if the content of the site is peer-reviewed. Peer-reviewed means that recognized practitioners or experts in the field have reviewed and judged the material to be valid and legitimate, and suitable for posting on the site. In order for information to be judged valid, it must have met certain scientific requirements and be recognized in the scientific literature (e.g. journals, textbooks, oral presentations at conferences).

SpineUniverse.com is one of the leading, award-winning educational spine sites with a diverse and talented editorial board. The site is rich in content including papers, videos, graphic artwork, and depictions of anatomy. There is a Community Section where patients can post their questions about spinal disorders. These questions are answered each day.

Other reputable sites include SRS.com, AAOS.org, WebMD.com, iscoliosis.com, Neurosurgery.org, NASS.com, Spine.org, Medem.com, Spine-Health.com, and others. Currently the most trust-worthy source of advice would come from your treating physician. Internet-savvy physicians should be able to point a patient in the right direction to find legitimate and useful spine-related sites.

Free Literature Search Engines
Patients can also make use of free literature search engines. Though some sites require payment of a registration fee, many are free to the public. These sites allow you to type in a "keyword" such as "disc herniation," "back pain," "lumbar spondylolisthesis," and search the professional peer-reviewed journals for pertinent scientific publications.

One should keep in mind, however, that these publications are for professionals and the text will be difficult to interpret by the layperson (patient). One may have to ask their physician for interpretation of articles that are found. Articles may be available in abbreviated (abstract) form, or they may be available in full length. Popular free sites include Medline (on Medscape.com), PubMed, National Institute of Health (NIH.gov), GratefulMed, and others.

Near Future: Patient-Physician Interaction
Soon the Internet will become useful for many of the patient-physician interactions that normally would take place in person, over the phone, via written mail, or via facsimile (FAX).

It is likely that most referrals and requests for appointments will be made via electronic mail. Patients will request and receive an appointment date and time via email.

Instead of receiving preliminary informational material via snail mail or at the initial office visit, patients will likely receive all information about the office location, telephone and fax numbers, and email addresses, the physician's professional background, and services offered all via email.

Patients will be able to send in information about their past medical and surgical history ahead of time and have it already reviewed and available at the time of their visit. Referring physicians will be able to send pertinent information and test results electronically, allowing for instant communication rather than relying upon the limitations of FAX and paper mail.

Electronic communication will likely expedite the communication of test results and treatment options to patients. Everyone has experienced waiting for a physician's office to call back with blood test or x-ray study results. Phone calls are often missed during everyone's busy daily schedule. Electronic communication offers both the physician and patient the capability to send questions and information when convenient.

Many physicians have been hesitant to use electronic communication because they fear that an unanswered message or inappropriate use of electronic communication (e.g. for an urgent matter) will result in litigation. Recent studies have shown, however, that both physicians and patients have been very satisfied with initial trials of electronic communication.

Security and Confidentiality
One of the main concerns about using the Internet and electronic communication (email) involves security and confidentiality. Computer hackers will always be able to break software security defenses,

and considerable time and effort is being spent to develop more secure transmission of patient medical information. It is likely that patients and physicians will be confident and comfortable exchanging patient-specific data electronically in the future.

Professional Development
The Internet is becoming increasingly useful to physicians for professional information and development.

All scientific spine organizations (e.g. North American Spine Society, American Association Neurosurgeons/ Congress of Neurological Surgeons Joint Section on Disorders of the Spine, Scoliosis Research Society, American Association of Orthopedic Surgery, Congress of Neurological Surgeons, American Association of Neurological Surgeons, GICD) now have websites that allow spine specialists to identify upcoming meetings and continuing medical education opportunities, new scientific reports and discoveries, new Food and Drug Administration (FDA) rulings, changes in reimbursement and coding issues, and other socioeconomic and legal news.

Furthermore, almost all scientific journals are now available on-line to professional subscribers (and some to the general public). Some journals are now only Internet-based (no paper journal is ever printed).

Practice Management
Physicians now can benefit from various sites that offer information and advice about practice management. Rather than hire an expensive business consultant, many private or academic spine groups can obtain useful information about office management including medical record retrieval, office visit protocol, human resource management, billing, and collections.

This will translate into a more efficient, productive visit for the patient when they seek the advice of a spine specialist.

Patient Education
Many physicians have used the Internet extensively to educate their patients *after* the initial examination. When a patient is told their diagnosis and treatment options, they can now be referred to several sites that allow them to read and educate themselves about their diagnosis and what to expect.

This easily accessible source of information will better prepare the patient to ask further questions and to be in more control of their health. A better-informed patient is more confident and more capable in making decisions with their consulting physician.

Summary
In summary, the Internet and electronic communication provide a powerful and convenient source of information for patients and physicians. Patients surfing the Internet for information must be discerning and should seek advice from their physician.

The most valid information comes from websites that are run by physicians, edited by physicians, and where the content is judged, critiqued, and published by physicians. Biased or incorrect information can be dangerous and invaluable to patients and physicians alike.

Patients will need to learn to discern between science and advertisement, between fact and fiction. Many fringe or quack treatments are advertised on the Internet. If they are not supported by published scientific information, then they are likely not yet part of standard practice.

Recognized professional organizations and journals, and peer-reviewed and edited spine sites offer the most reliable and valid information. Most physicians are more than happy to offer their advice regarding information that their patients find on the Internet.

The best-educated patient is the patient most confident and able to manage their spinal condition.

Figure 1: Spinal Column

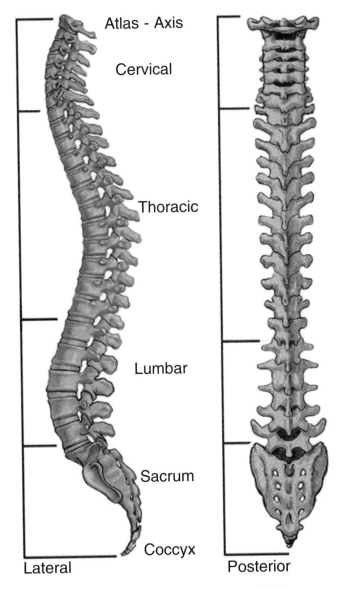

Atlas - Axis

Cervical

Thoracic

Lumbar

Sacrum

Coccyx

Lateral

Posterior

Figure 2: Atlas - Axis

Atlas

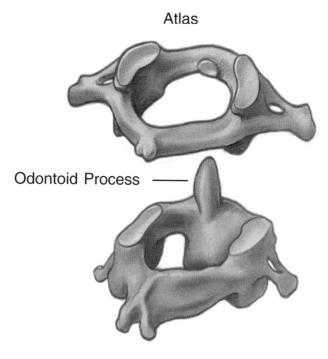

Odontoid Process ——

Axis

Figure 3: Vertebral Segment

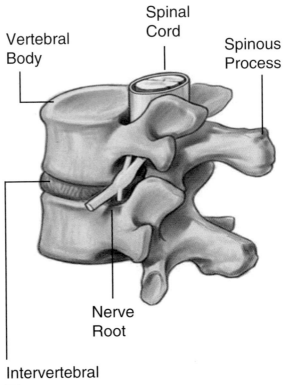

Vertebral Body

Spinal Cord

Spinous Process

Nerve Root

Intervertebral Disc

Figure 4: Intervertebral Disc

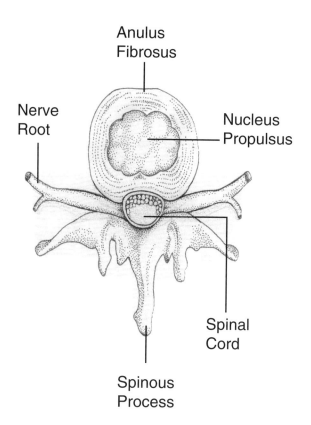

Anulus
Fibrosus

Nerve
Root

Nucleus
Propulsus

Spinal
Cord

Spinous
Process

Figure 5: Facet Joints

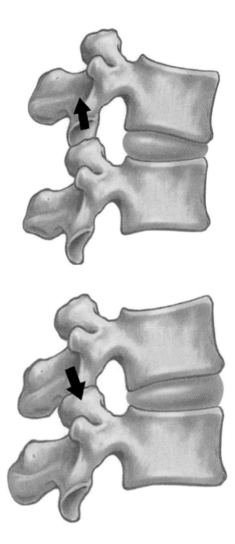

Figure 6: Spinal Cord Meninges

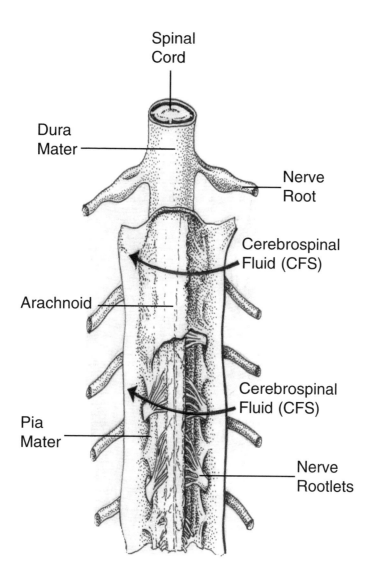

Spinal Cord

Dura Mater

Nerve Root

Cerebrospinal Fluid (CFS)

Arachnoid

Cerebrospinal Fluid (CFS)

Pia Mater

Nerve Rootlets

Figure 7: Spinal Nerves

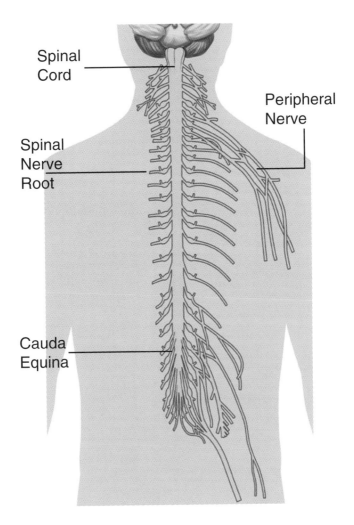

Spinal Cord

Peripheral Nerve

Spinal Nerve Root

Cauda Equina

Figure 8: Ligaments

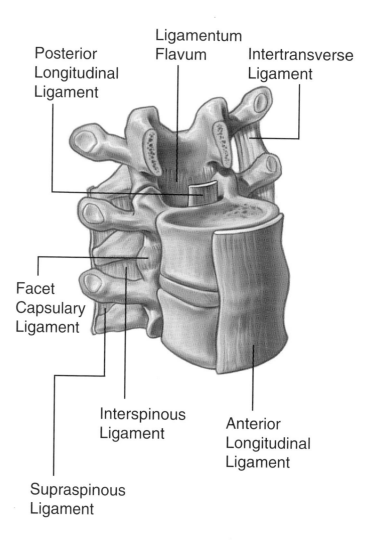

Posterior Longitudinal Ligament

Ligamentum Flavum

Intertransverse Ligament

Facet Capsulary Ligament

Interspinous Ligament

Anterior Longitudinal Ligament

Supraspinous Ligament

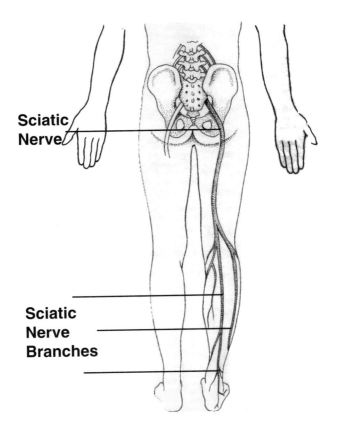

Sciatic
Nerve

Sciatic
Nerve
Branches

Figure 10: Vertebral Fracture

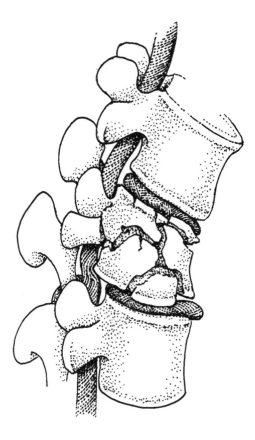

Figure 11: Spondylolisthesis

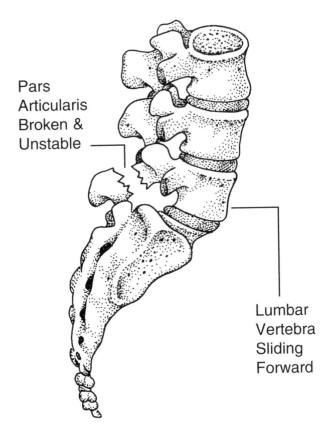

Pars
Articularis
Broken &
Unstable

Lumbar
Vertebra
Sliding
Forward

Figure 12: Scoliosis

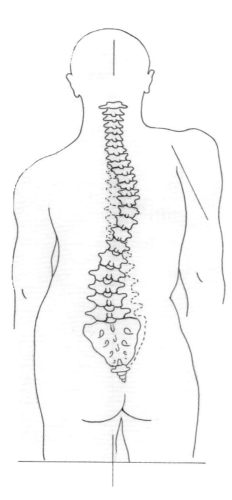

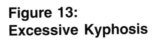

Figure 13:
Excessive Kyphosis

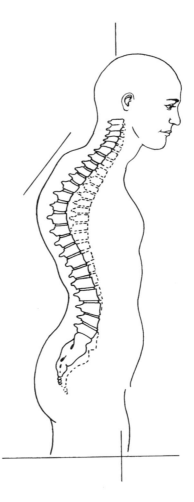

**Figure 14:
Excessive Lordosis**

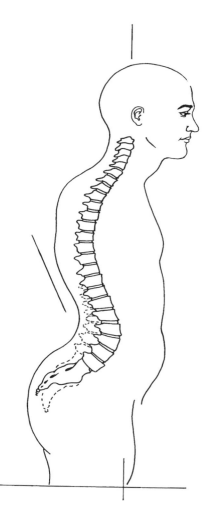

Figure 15: Degenerative Disorders

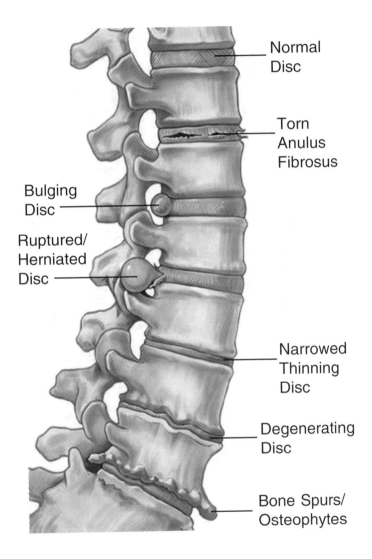

Normal Disc

Torn Anulus Fibrosus

Bulging Disc

Ruptured/ Herniated Disc

Narrowed Thinning Disc

Degenerating Disc

Bone Spurs/ Osteophytes

Figure 16: Spinal Stenosis

A 'window' is used to illustrate the neuroforamen - pathways through which the nerve roots exit the spinal canal.

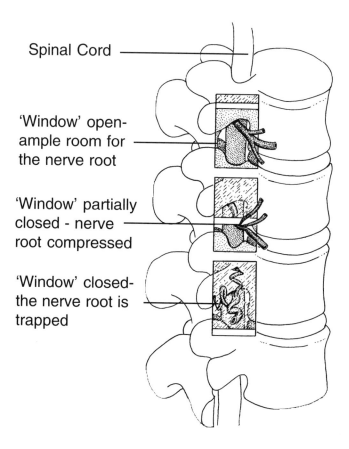

Spinal Cord

'Window' open-ample room for the nerve root

'Window' partially closed - nerve root compressed

'Window' closed-the nerve root is trapped

Figure 17: Osteoporosis

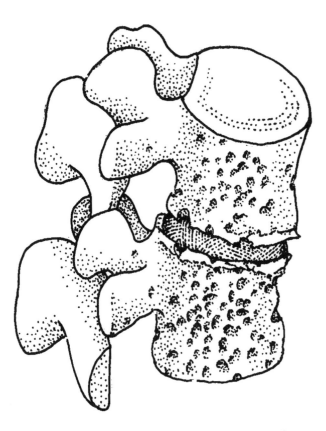

The vertebral bodies have lost density or strength. The porous, weak bone is susceptible to fracture and collapse

Figure 18: Proper Posture

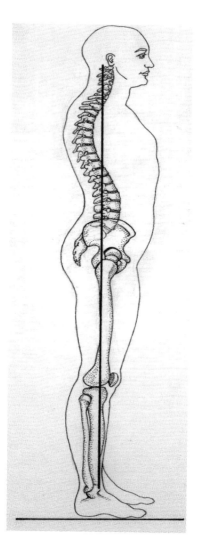

Figure 19: Minimally Invasive Spine Surgery - thru "Portals"

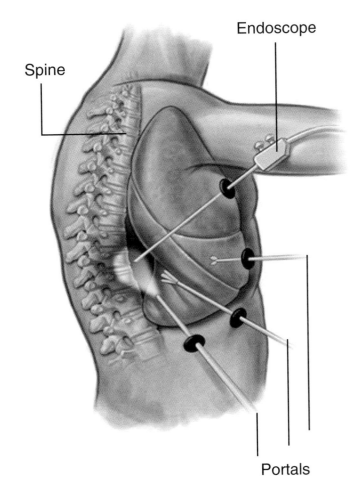

Endoscope

Spine

Portals

Figure 20: Interbody Cage

Vertebra

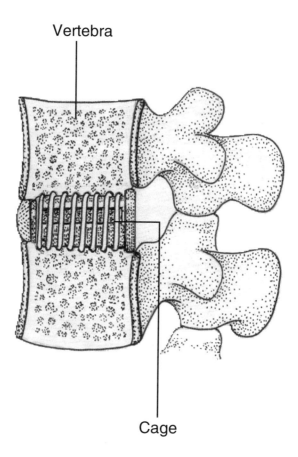

Cage

Figure 21a: Laminotomy

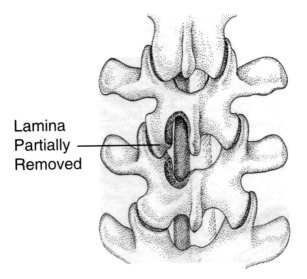

Lamina Partially Removed

Figure 21b: Laminectomy

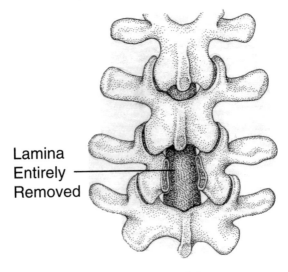

Lamina Entirely Removed

Posterior View

Figure 22: Instrumentation and Fusion

Vertebra

Disc

Screw

Bone Graft

Rod

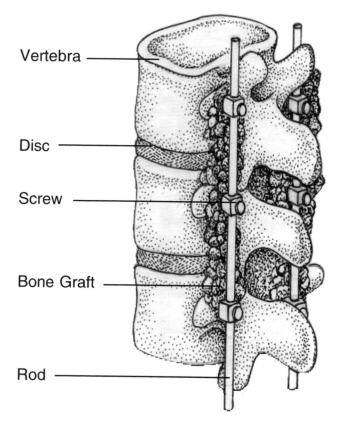

Glossary of Terms and
Easy Pronunciation Guide

ACUPUNCTURE (ak-u-punk-chur) Practitioner inserts special needles into the body at specific points to control pain and restore inner harmony.

ACUTE PAIN (ah-cute) Severe or sharp pain that may follow injury or surgery. This type of pain is short-term.

ADRENAL HORMONE (ah-dre-null) Estrogen is a hormone produced by the adrenal gland and is needed for healthy bones.

ALLOGRAFT (al-o-graft) Donor bone.

ANALGESIC (an-all-jee-sik) Medication to control pain.

ANESTHESIOLOGIST (an-es-thee-z-al-oh-jist) Physician who administers sedatives and pain medication during a surgical procedure.

ANKYLOSING SPONDYLITIS
(an-key-low-sing spon-dee-lie-tis) Chronic and progressive inflammatory disease affecting the spinal joints.

ANKYLOSIS (an-key-low-sis) Disease that causes the spine to lose flexibility and stiffen.

ANTERIOR (an-tear-e-or) Front.

ANTERIOR LONGITUDINAL LIGAMENT
(an-tear-e-or lon-ji-tude-in-al) Spinal ligament that attaches to the front of each vertebra.

ANTI-DEPRESSANT (anti-dee-press-ant) Prescription drug used to alleviate depression and anxiety.

ANTI-INFLAMMATORY (anti-in-flam-ah-tory)
Drug used to reduce swelling and inflammation.

ANULUS FIBROSUS (an-you-lus fye-bro-sis)
Tough tire-like outer layer of a vertebral disc.

ARACHNOID (ah-rack-noid) One of the protective membranes covering the spinal cord.

ARTHROPATHY (arth-row-pathy) Joint disorder.

ARTHRITIS (arth-rye-tis)
Common joint disease causing inflammation and pain.

ARTICULATE (ar-tick-you-late) Move, such as a joint.

AUTOGRAFT (auto-graft)
Bone taken from the patient's body used in fusion.

BONE DENSITY SCAN - Diagnostic imaging tool that measures the density of bone.

BONE GRAFT
Harvested bone used in spinal fusion procedures.

BONE STIMULATOR
Device that stimulates bones to heal or grow.

BONY OVERGROWTH or BONE SPUR
Abnormal growth of bone; also called an osteophyte.

BRACE - Custom-fitted, removable support, worn to stabilize the spine.

BULGING DISC - The anulus of a vertebral disc protrudes with the nucleus pulposus intact. Also known as a Contained Disc.

CAGE - Specific type of spinal device used in some types of instrumentation and fusion procedures to fill empty disc space.

CALCIFICATION (kals-see-fi-cay-shun)
Body process that causes bone to harden.

CALLUS - Granular material the body produces and deposits at the site of a fracture to help mending.

CANCELLOUS (cancel-lus)
Interior compartment of bone resembling latticework.

CANNULA (can-u-lah) Small metal tube used during percutaneous and laser procedures through which small surgical instruments are passed.

CARTILAGE (car-ti-ledge)
Smooth coating covering (bonded to) joint surfaces.

CARTILAGINOUS (car-t-lay-gin-us)
Relating to cartilage.

CAUDA EQUINA (caw-dah e-kwhy-nah) Lower end of the spinal cord near the first lumbar vertebra; resembles the tail of a horse.

CAUSALGIA (cause-al-gee-ah) Severe pain that usually follows injury to a peripheral nerve.

CEREBROSPINAL FLUID (sir-ee-bro-spinal) Liquid cushion within the layers of the spinal cord.

CERVICAL SPINE (sir-ve-kal) First seven vertebrae starting at the base of the skull abbreviated C1, C2, C3, C4, C5, C6, and C7.

CHRONIC PAIN
Continuous pain described as mild to severe.

CLAUSTROPHOBIC (claw-stro-foe-bick)
Fear of being in an enclosed place.

CLINICAL SYMPTOMS
Symptoms that define a particular disease.

COCCYX (cock-six) Last bone formation below the sacrum; also called the tailbone.

COLLAGEN (call-ah-gin)
Protein manufactured by the body; mends fracture.

COMPRESSION FRACTURE
Fracture that may cause a vertebra to collapse.

COMPRESSIVE NEUROPATHY (ner-row-path-ee)
Pressure on nerves that may cause swelling and pain.

COMPUTERIZED AXIAL TOMOGRAPHY - Abbreviated CT Scan or CAT Scan. Diagnostic imaging tool that utilizes multiple x-ray beams to produce detailed slices of anatomy.

CONGENITAL - Present at birth; such as a disorder.

CONTAINED DISC - Also called a Bulging Disc.

CORPECTOMY (core-peck-toe-me) Surgical removal of bone from the front of the neck (cervical spine).

CORTICAL (core-tea-cul)
Outer layer of bone resembling concentric rings.

DEGENERATIVE DISC DISEASE (DDD) - Biochemical changes associated with aging that may cause discs to crack, become thin, bulge, or herniate.

DERMATOME (dur-ma-tome) - Specific area of skin supplied by fibers of a single nerve root.

DIAGNOSIS - Name of a particular disorder.

DISC (or disk) Also called an Intervertebral Disc. Cushion-like shock absorber located between two vertebrae.

DISCECTOMY (dis-eck-toe-me) Surgical removal of a portion of or an entire intervertebral disc.

DISCOGRAPHY (dis-ah-gra-fee) Specific type of x-ray used to reveal the pathology of a disc.

DURA MATER (doo-rah-matter) One of the protective membranes covering the spinal cord.

DYSESTHESIA (dis-ah-thee-z-ah)
Abnormal or unpleasant sensation.

ELECTRICAL STIMULATION (TENS) - Also called Transcutaneous Electrical Stimulation, (TENS). Modality used to stimulate circulation, alleviate swelling, pain, and enhance healing.

ELECTROCARDIOGRAM(electro-car-dee-oh-gram) (ECG) Test used to take an electrical picture of the heart.

ELECTROMYOGRAPHY (elec-tro-my-ah-gra-fee) (EMG)
Test used to determine if muscle function is normal.

ENDOSCOPE (en-doe-scope) Surgical instrument used
to examine the inside of the body via a tube.

EPIDURAL (ep-e-do-ral) Injection into the spinal canal's
epidural space to help alleviate pain.

EPIDURAL SPACE (ep-e-do-ral) Space above and
surrounding the dura mater of the spinal cord.

FACET JOINT (fah-set) Joints in the spine.

FASCIA (fay-sha) Fibrous sheets that encase muscles.

FIBROCARTILAGE (fybro-car-til-ledge)
Super strong cartilage.

FLUOROSCOPIC GUIDANCE (floor-o-skop-ik)
Imaging tool used during surgery.

FLUOROSCOPE (floor-o-scope)
X-ray equipment used in fluoroscopy.

FORAMEN (foe-ray-men)
Space where a nerve root exits the spinal canal.

FORAMINAL STENOSIS (foe-ray-min-al sten-oh-sis)
Narrowing or closing of a spinal foramen.

FORAMINOTOMY (for-am-not-toe-me) Surgical
procedure used to increase the size of the foramen.

GENERAL ANESTHESIA (an-es-thee-z-ah) Drugs used
by an anesthesiologist during surgery that temporarily
disable nerve impulses making the patient unconscious
and pain free.

HARDWARE - Slang term for instrumentation. Refers to cages, plates, rods, and screws used in surgical procedures to stabilize the spine.

HAVERSIAN SPACES (hav-er-sh-on)
Vascular canals in bone.

HERNIATED DISC (her-knee-ate-ed) Non-Contained Disc; the anulus breaks open allowing the nucleus pulposus to leak out of the disc.

HYPERALGESIA (hi-per-al-gee-zee-ah)
Increased sensitivity to pain.

HYPERESTHESIA (hi-per-es-thee-zee-ah)
Acute abnormal skin sensitivity.

HYPEREXTENSION (hi-per ex-ten-shun)
Extension of a joint/soft tissue beyond normal limits.

HYPERFLEXION (hi-per flex-un)
Flexion of a joint/soft tissue beyond normal limits.

HYPERREFLEXIA (hi-per-re-flex-e-ah)
Condition causing deep tendon reflexes to become exaggerated.

HYPOALGESIA (hi-poe-al-g-zee-ah)
Diminished skin sensation.

IDIOPATHIC SCOLIOSIS
(id-dee-oh-path-ick sko-lee-oh-sis)
Abnormal curvature of the spine for which the cause is unknown.

INFLAMMATION (in-flah-may-shun) Swelling.

INFORMED CONSENT - Document the patient signs following full disclosure of a medical procedure.

INTERSPINOUS LIGAMENT (in-ter-spy-nus)
See ligament.

INTERTRANSVERSE LIGAMENT (in-ter-tranz-verse)
See ligament.

KYPHOSIS (kye-foe-sis) Abnormal forward curving of the spine; may cause a hump to form in the shoulder blade area of the upper back. Opposite condition: Lordosis.

KYPHOTIC (kye-fah-tick) Relating to kyphosis.

LAMINA (lamb-in-ah) Thin bony plate that protects the spinal canal.

LAMINAE (lamb-in-e) Plural of lamina.

LAMINECTOMY (lamb-in-eck-toe-me)
Surgical removal of the lamina.

LAMINOTOMY (lamb-in-ah-toe-me)
Surgical removal of a portion of the lamina.

LASER (lay-zer) Surgical tool that uses an infrared source to divide or destroy tissue.

LIGAMENT (lig-ah-ment) Strong fibrous connective tissue that links bone, cartilages or other structures together.

LIGAMENTUM FLAVUM (lig-ah-men-tum flay-vum)
Yellow colored ligament that connects the laminae to two adjacent vertebrae.

LOCAL ANESTHETIC (local an-es-thet-ick)
Injection at or near the procedure site to block pain impulses.

LORDOSIS (lor-doe-sis)
Abnormal inward curving of the spine; also called swayback. Opposite condition: Kyphosis.

LORDOTIC (lor-dot-ick) Relating to lordosis.

LUMBAR SPINE (lum-bar) Five (or six) vertebrae that follow the last thoracic vertebra abbreviated L1, L2, L3, L4, and L5.

MAGNETIC RESONANCE IMAGING (MRI) Imaging tool that produces detailed pictures without radiation.

MARROW - Semi-soft center of bone responsible for production of red blood cells.

MENINGES (men-in-jez) Protective layers covering the spinal cord.

METASTASIZE (ma-taz-ta-size) When disease spreads to another part of the body such as cancer.

MICRODISCECTOMY (mycro-dis-eck-toe-me) Surgical removal of a part of or an entire vertebral disc using microscopic magnification.

MODALITY (mow-dal-it-tee) Passive treatment or therapy that does not require patient participation.

MUSCLE SPASM - Involuntary contraction of one or more muscles; may cause pain.

MYELOPATHY (my-il-lop-ah-thee)
Disorder or dysfunction of the spinal cord.

MYOFASCIAL RELEASE (my-oh-fash-e-al)
Local massage to manipulate the muscle fascia.

NARCOTIC - Prescription drug to control pain.

NERVE BLOCK - Type of injection into or around a nerve or group of nerves that blocks the passage of pain impulses.

NERVE CONDUCTION VELOCITY (NCV) Sensitive test that determines a nerve's ability to transmit an impulse.

NEURALGIA (nu-ral-g-al)
Nerve pain caused by damage or dysfunction.

NEURITIS (nu-ry-tis)
Inflammation of one or more nerves.

NEUROFORAMEN (nu-row for-a-men) Small openings in the spine that provide space for nerve roots to exit the spinal canal.

NEUROPATHY (nu-rop-ah-thee) Inflammatory process involving nerves. This type of pain is called neuropathic pain.

NEUTRAL SPINE - Denotes good posture. The spine is not subjected to unnecessary stress.

NOCICEPTIVE (no-si-sep-tiv) Response to a painful stimulus. Localized pain.

NON-CONTAINED DISC - See Herniated Disc.

NUCLEUS PULPOSUS (new-klee-us pul-poe-sis)
Gel-like center of a vertebral disc.

ODONTOID PROCESS (oh-don-toyed)
Tooth-like projection from the axis.

OPIOID or OPIATE (oh-pe-oid or oh-pe-ate)
Drug chemically related to opium; used to treat pain.

OSSIFICATION (os-e-fik-kay-shun)
Formation of bone.

OSTEOARTHRITIS (OA) (os-t-o-arth-rye-tis)
Degenerative form of arthritis.

OSTEOBLAST (os-t-o-blast) Bone forming cell.

OSTEOCLAST (os-t-o-klast)
Large cell that absorbs and removes bone.

OSTEOPHYTE (os-t-o-fight)
Outward growth of bone; also called a bone spur.

OSTEOPOROSIS (os-t-o-pour-o-sis) Disease that causes bones to lose density and become susceptible to fracture.

OUTPATIENT SURGERY – Same day surgery.

PALPATION (pal-pay-shun)
Procedure to examine the body by touch.

PARALYSIS (pa-ral-eh-sis)
Loss of function, inability to move.

PARESTHESIA (par-s-thee-z-ah) Abnormal sensations such as tingling or pins and needles.

PARS ARTICULARIS (parz are-tick-you-lar-es)
Part of the posterior vertebra, including the facet joints that attach to the vertebral body.

PATIENT-CONTROLLED ANALGESIA (PCA)
Controlled pumping device that allows post-operative patients to self-dose pain relieving medication.

PEDICLE - Bony process that projects backward from the vertebra connecting the lamina on either side.

PERCUTANEOUS SURGERY (per-cue-tay-nee-us)
Surgical procedure performed through a small hole made in the skin.

PERIPHERAL NEUROPATHY
(pe-rif-er-al nu-rop-ah-thee) Disease affecting the nerves branching into the extremities.

PHYSICAL THERAPY - Conservative treatment that may include ice/heat, electrical stimulation, massage, ultrasound, and exercise.

PIA MATER (pee-ah matter)
One of the layers that protects the spinal cord.

POSTERIOR - Rear, behind.

POSTERIOR LONGITUDINAL LIGAMENT
Spinal ligament that runs vertically and behind the vertebrae to reinforce the intervertebral discs.

RADIATE (ray-dee-ate) Pain or sensation that travels away from the point of origin.

RADICULOPATHY (rah-dick-u-lop-ah-thee)
Pain caused by injury to a nerve root.

RADIOGRAPH - X-ray.

RECOVERY ROOM - Area supervised by medical personnel where a patient is taken immediately following surgery.

REFERRED PAIN - Pain felt in a part of the body separate from the origin of the pain.

RHEUMATOID ARTHRITIS (RA)
(room-ah-toyed arth-rye-tis) Progressive form of arthritis that may be painfully destructive.

ROOTLET (root-let)
Nerve root that shoots off from the spinal cord.

RUPTURED DISC - See Herniated Disc.

SACRAL (say-kral) Relating to the sacrum.

SACROILIAC (say-kro-ill-e-ak)
Relating to the sacrum such as the sacroiliac joint.

SACRUM (say-krum) - Triangular shaped bone mass located below the last lumbar vertebra.

SCIATICA (sy-attic-ka) Compressive or inflammatory process involving the sciatic nerve.

SCOLIOSIS (sko-lee-oh-sis) Disease that causes the spine to curve abnormally to the side in the shape of an "S" or "C."

SEDATIVE - Medication administered to calm the patient or to induce sleep.

SENSORY - Physical feeling such as touch.

SLIPPED DISC - An erroneous term used to mean bulging or herniated disc.

SOFT TISSUE INJURY - Injury to tendons, ligaments, or muscles.

SPINAL FUSION and SPINAL INSTRUMENTATION Surgical procedures using bone graft and cages, plates, rods, and screws to stabilize the spine.

SPINAL MENINGITIS (men-in-ji-tis) Serious infection causing inflammation of the membranes in the brain and/or spinal cord.

SPINAL STENOSIS (spinal sten-oh-sis) Narrowing or closing of the neuroforamen causing nerve root compression and pain.

SPINAL TUMOR – Rare abnormal growth; either benign or malignant (cancerous).

SPONDYLOLISTHESIS (spon-de-low-lis-thee-sis) Disorder caused by one vertebra slipping over the vertebra below.

SPONDYLOSIS (spon-dee-low-sis) Degenerative disease that may affect both the disc and the facet joints.

SPRAIN or STRAIN - Hyperextension or hyperflexion disorder caused by the extension of a joint or soft tissue beyond normal limits.

SUPRASPINOUS LIGAMENT (sue-pra-spine-us) See ligament.

SYNOVIAL FLUID (si-no-vee-al fluid) Fluid that lubricates and nourishes joints and cartilage.

TAILBONE - Last bone formation below the sacrum.

TENDON (ten-dun) Sturdy fibrous band of tissue that attaches muscle to bone.

THORACIC SPINE (thor-as-ick) 12 vertebrae following the last cervical vertebra abbreviated T1 through T12.

TRIGGER POINT INJECTION - Injection of pain relieving medication at the site of pain.

ULTRASOUND - Modality used to relax muscles by promoting deep warmth into soft tissues to increase local circulation and to enhance healing.

URINALYSIS (yu-ri-nal-is-sis) Test to analyze urine.

VERTEBRA (ver-ta-bra) Singular form.

VERTEBRAE (ver-ta-bray) Plural form.

VERTEBRAL (ver-tee-brawl) A specific vertebra. Bony elements of the spinal column totaling 33 vertebrae.

WHIPLASH - Intensive soft tissue neck injury.

X-RAY - Radiograph; a common diagnostic imaging tool that uses radiation to create a picture of a body part.

ZYGAPOPHYSEAL JOINTS (zye-gap-o-fiz-e-all)
See facet joints.

Index

Compressive neuropathy 42, 169
Congenital disorders 50, 53, 169
Contained, non-contained 49, 146-147, 158,
      165, 169, 175
Corpectomy 91, 169
CT Scan 34, 36, 54, 116, 169
Curves 23, 48-49, 161

Degenerative Disc Disease (DDD) 54-55, 158, 170
Degenerative disorders 50-57, 81-102, 158, 170
Dermatomes 26, 170
Diagnostic tests 33-38, 89, 94-95, 100
Discectomy 43, 77, 96-97, 103-114, 170
Discography 37, 170
Disc 23-25, 54-55, 83-84, 146-147, 158, 165 170
Dura mater 26, 149, 170

Electrical stimulation (TENS) 124, 170
Electromyography (EMG) 37, 94-95, 171
Endplate 25
Epidural steroid injection 60-61, 67-68, 96, 171
Exercise 57, 120, 124, 126-127, 135
Extensor 27

Facet joint 25, 47, 61, 68, 83-84, 98,
      100-101, 148, 171
Fascia 27, 171
Fluoroscopy 60, 67-68, 106, 115, 171
Foramen, foramina 26, 47, 53-55, 60, 159, 171
Foraminal stenosis 42, 53-54, 159, 171
Foraminotomy 47, 78, 171
Forward flexor 27
Fracture 45-46, 55, 153, 169
Fusion, cage 77-79, 91-92, 163, 165, 168, 179

Haversian space 23, 172
Heat 124-125
Herniated disc 42, 49-50, 61, 77, 81-82, 85,
        93-97, 158, 172
Hydrotherapy 125
Hyperextension 41, 172
Hyperflexion 41, 172

Ice 124-125

Image-guided spine surgery 80, 115-116
Infection 44, 81, 87
Informed consent 71-72, 173
Injection 47, 59-62, 67-68, 100-101
Instrumentation, hardware 78-79, 115-119,
        163, 165, 172, 179
Internet 137-143
Intersegmental system 26
Interspinous ligament 26, 151, 173
Intertransverse ligament 26, 151
Intervertebral disc 24-25, 55, 83-84, 146, 158
Intradiscal Electrothermoplasty (IDET) 62-63
Intrasegmental system 26

Kyphotic, kyphosis 23, 48-49, 56, 156, 173

Laboratory tests 38
Laminectomy 77, 106, 164, 173
Laminotomy 43, 77, 97, 164, 173
Lateral flexor 27
Leg pain 42-43, 47, 53-54, 60, 103
Ligament 26-27, 39, 151, 173
Ligamentum flavum 26, 151, 173
Lordotic, lordosis 23, 49, 157, 174
Lumbar 24, 42, 53-54, 103-114, 174

Osteoclast 23, 176
Osteocyte 23
Osteophyte 52, 158, 176
Osteoporosis 20, 36, 46, 55-57, 160, 176

Pain assessment 66
Pain diagram 30
Pain management 58-68, 129-136
Pain, acute, chronic 29, 30, 58-59, 86-87,
        166, 169
Palpate 31, 176
Patient-Controlled Analgesia (PCA) 63-64, 74, 177
Peripheral nerve block 61
Peripheral Nervous System (PNS) 26-27, 61, 150
Peripheral neuropathy 43, 177
Physical examination 29-31
Physical therapy 41, 47, 59, 62, 67, 96, 110,
        120-128, 161, 177
Pia mater 26, 149, 177
Posterior longitudinal ligament 27, 151, 177
Post-operative pain 63-64, 74, 92
Posture 120-128, 161
Pre-operative 72-73

Radiculopathy 93-96, 103, 177
Radiofrequency discal nucleoplasty 63
Range of motion 31-32, 94
Recovery 74, 92-93, 108-110, 178
Rheumatoid Arthritis (RA) 52, 81, 87, 178
Rotator 27

Sacrum 24, 52, 104, 178
Sciatica, sciatic nerve 42-43, 103-104, 152, 178
Scoliosis, idiopathic 19, 48, 155, 172, 178
Slipped disc 42, 49-50, 158, 179

. . . .*Notes*. . . . .

. . . .*Notes*. . . . .

. . . . .Notes. . . . .

ORDER FORM

Save Your Aching Back and Neck,
A Patient's Guide

Postal Orders: SYA Press and Research, Inc.
5694 Mission Center Road #294
San Diego, CA 92108-4380

On-Line Orders: http://www.spineuniverse.com

Name _____

Company Name _____

Address _____

City _____

State _____ Zip _____

Telephone _____

Fax _____

How many copies?
($16.95/copy)

Sales Tax (CA only)

Shipping/Handling $4.55
(USPO Priority)

Total Enclosed

. . . . .Notes. . . . .